Midwifery
Practice
A research-based approach

Ed

Jo Alexand   *alerie Levy*
and *Sarah Roch*

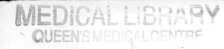
© Series: Jo Alexander, Valerie Levy & Sarah Roch

© This volume: Communication in midwifery, Mavis Kirkham;
Iron and vitamin supplementation during pregnancy,
Elsa Montgomery; Exercise and pregnancy, Gillian Halksworth;
Fetal medicine, Joanne Whelton; The elderly primigravida,
Louise Silverton; Couvade – the retaliation of marginalised
fathers, Paul Summersgill; Safer motherhood – a midwifery
challenge, Mary Kensington; Pain and the neonate, Valerie
Fletcher; Workload measurement in midwifery, Jean Ball;
Negligence litigation research and the practice of midwifery,
Robert Dingwall.

First published 1993 by
THE MACMILLAN PRESS LTD
Houndmills, Basingstoke, Hampshire RG21 2XS
and London
Companies and representatives
throughout the world

ISBN 0–333–57617–9

A catalogue record for this book is available
from the British Library

Typeset by Footnote Graphics,
Warminster, Wiltshire

Printed in China

Dedicated to

ANN STEWART

Midwifery Professional Officer and Adviser
English National Board for Nursing,
Midwifery and Health Visiting 1983–1991

In memory of an outstanding midwife
who encouraged greatly the development
of research-based practice in midwifery

Contents

Other volumes in the Midwifery Practice series

Contributors to this volume

Jean A Ball MSc DipN RGN RM
Senior Teaching Fellow, Nuffield Institute for Health Services Studies, the University of Leeds
Jean Ball has written widely on aspects of nursing and midwifery management, especially topics relating to quality assurance and staffing levels. As well as her previous management posts, she was formerly Director of Research for North Lincolnshire Health Authority. She contributed the Foreword to Volume 3 in this series.

Robert Dingwall MA PhD
Professor and Head of the School of Social Studies, University of Nottingham
Robert Dingwall is a sociologist who has worked in both medical and legal fields. Before his appointment to the University of Nottingham, he worked at the Universities of Aberdeen and Oxford on a variety of projects including studies of health visitor training, agency decision making in child abuse, the social history of nursing and midwifery and the impact of medical negligence litigation.

Valerie Fletcher MSc RGN SCM HV
Neonatal Midwife, Paediatric Department, Glasgow Royal Maternity Hospital
Valerie Fletcher is an experienced neonatal nurse and midwife whose own research has alerted her to potential problems in the way babies are perceived and treated in neonatal intensive care units.

Gillian Halksworth BA(Hons) RGN RM
Integrated Midwife, Taff Ely, Mid Glamorgan
Gillian Halksworth works as a team member, providing continuity of care for midwifery clients. Her brief currently includes teaching aquanatal classes. In 1991, she was awarded a scholarship which facilitated travelling abroad to observe midwifery services. She is currently studying for a masters degree and has a particular interest in social deprivation and pregnancy outcome.

Mary Kensington BA RGN RM ADM
Formerly Midwifery Sister, Maternity Department, Odstock Hospital, Salisbury
Since writing this chapter, Mary Kensington has returned to her native New Zealand. Her previous work experience, in a number of different countries including Australia, Northern Canada and Thailand, has given her a global perspective on health issues and maternity care.

Mavis J Kirkham PhD SRN SCM Cert Ed
Principal Lecturer in Midwifery, De Montford University, Leicester
An internationally respected author, researcher and practitioner, Mavis Kirkham is well known for her work on midwives' communication skills. She lectures widely on reseach in midwifery.

Elsa Montgomery BSc(Hons) RGN RM
Midwife, Princess Anne Hospital, Southampton
Elsa Montgomery's current post, that of a staff midwife rotating through all departments, keeps her in touch with all aspects of 'grass roots' midwifery. She wrote this chapter while on maternity leave.

Louise I Silverton BSc SRN SCM MSc MTD
The Nightingale and Guy's College of Health, London
An experienced midwife teacher, Louise Silverton is currently Head of Maternal and Child Health. She has carried out research into breastfeeding, and has a particular interest in ethics relating to midwifery practice.

Paul R Summersgill BA(Hons) PGCE
Department of Nursing Studies, Faculty of Medicine, the University of Southampton
A sociologist by training, Paul Summersgill now lectures in his subject to midwives and nurses. His interest in the role of fathers in the childbearing process is personal as well as academic (as he is a father himself). He is currently working for his PhD.

Joanne Whelton RN RM Dip Counselling Skills
Regional Co-ordinator, Confidential Enquiry into Stillbirths and Deaths in Infancy (CESDI)
Joanne Whelton is now based at the London Hospital Medical College at Queen Mary's, Westminster. She has studied the understanding and application of research (ENB course 870) and has written a number of articles focusing on the sensitive dilemmas arising from prenatal testing and fetal medicine.

Foreword

I am delighted to write the foreword to a new volume in the series *Midwifery Practice: a research-based approach*. The success of the three previous volumes dealing with antenatal, intrapartum and postnatal care reflects the interest and enthusiasm that exists amongst midwives both about research itself and about its relevance to their everyday practice.

This volume has been written with a view to exploring various aspects of midwifery practice from the use of iron and vitamin supplements in pregnancy through to the management of pain in the neonate and then highlighting the challenges that exist for the midwife in ensuring that her practice stands up to research scrutiny. The 'Practice checks' incorporated into the chapters should ensure that research findings are applied to care and delivery.

The contributors also address some of the more complex issues that may be encountered by the midwife. The recent developments in the field of fetal medicine are explored with interest and the reader is encouraged to consider the less comfortable areas into which consideration of such advances inevitably lead. The psychological and ethical issues that will be faced by parents and midwives in these situations are highlighted as is the midwife's need to prepare herself for such challenges.

With a distinguished list of contributors and a firm pragmatic base this volume complements the previous books in the series and provides an excellent resource for midwives as they seek to develop their practice, set their standards and audit their performance.

Ann Stewart to whom this book has been dedicated spent her professional life in the pursuit of excellence in midwifery practice and education. This book serves as a fitting tribute to her.

Joan Greenwood
Nursing Officer, Midwifery and Maternity Services, Department of Health

Preface

Since the publication of the first three volumes in this series, events have moved on apace. There has been a considerable increase in the scope of graduate education available for midwives, with the first MSc programmes in Midwifery Studies now in existence. Pre-registration midwifery courses now have to be validated at least to higher education diploma level and, following the UKCC decision in 1991, this will soon apply to all post-registration courses. These developments in higher education have probably sprung, at least in part, from an increasing recognition by the profession of the importance of underpinning practice with sound research and the resultant need for all midwives to be knowledgeable 'consumers' of research.

For those who venture to undertake research (who could be called research 'producers'), there is an increasing recognition of the need for specific preparation for this work, and the development of a diploma course in research methods is a welcome initiative. All 'products' have to be distributed and important advances have taken place in this field also. In 1990, the first of what are to be annual publications of MIRIAD (the Midwifery Research Database) took place. MIRIAD has made available a wealth of information about studies relevant to midwifery conducted in the United Kingdom, both completed and ongoing. It is produced by the Midwifery Research Initiative based at the National Perinatal Epidemiology Unit, Oxford, and is now distributed through the Royal College of Midwives. Another development facilitating the distribution of research information was the inauguration in 1991 of a new national 'Research in Midwifery Conference' which is also to become an annual event. The Midwives Information and Resource Service (MIDIRS), the Midwives, Research and Childbirth series of books and the Research and the Midwife Conference continue to make outstanding contributions to the dissemination of research information.

Despite these initiatives, research information is still not always easily accessible to midwives. Access to good library services may be difficult, particularly for midwives working at a distance from academic centres. Libraries are not always as well staffed as they might be and stocks of journals and other resources may be inadequate (Shepherd 1990). Searching the literature is always time consuming and photocopying often expensive.

This series is intended to help fill the vacuum which exists between the current state of research and the literature readily available to practitioners. The series offers midwives and student midwives a broad ranging survey and analysis of the research literature relating to central areas of clinical practice. We hope that it will also prove useful to childbearing women, their families and others involved with the maternity care services. The books do not intend to provide the comprehensive coverage of a definitive textbook; indeed their strength derives from the in-depth treatment of a selection of topics. The topic areas were chosen with care and authors (most, but not all, of whom are midwives) were approached who have particular research interest and expertise. On the basis of their critical appraisal of the literature, the authors make recommendations for clinical practice, and thus the predominant feature of these books is the link made between research and key areas of practice.

The chapters have a common structure, identical to that found in the three earlier volumes, and this is described below. We have been led to believe, from readers' and reviewers' comments, that the structure is useful and appropriate. Some knowledge of basic research terminology will prove useful but its lack should not discourage readers.

We owe a debt of gratitude to many people; most of all to our authors who have worked so painstakingly to produce their contributions, to our publishers and to the many practitioners and students who have made valuable comments on draft material. A most welcome development has been the invaluable part that Richenda Milton-Thompson has played as publisher's editor for this series. She joined our 'team' some way through the production of the first three volumes and has had a pivotal role in the preparation of this one. Her skill and quiet enthusiasm have greatly enhanced our enjoyment of this collaborative venture.

There is certainly no lack of potential material for this series. The recent House of Commons Health Committee Report (1992) endorsed the importance of midwifery research and also urged the Government to provide an unprecedented opportunity for midwives to regain their autonomy and provide holistic care for women and their families. The consequences of any changes in patterns of care resulting from this report, or indeed from other initiatives, will need careful investigation; the prospect of perhaps collating information from these studies in further volumes is an exciting one.

JA
VL
SR
November 1992

■ Common structure of chapters

In fulfilment of the aims of the series, each chapter follows a common structure:

1. The introduction offers a digest of the contents;

2. '*It is assumed that you are already aware of the following...*' establishes the prerequisite knowledge and experience assumed of the reader;

3. The main body of the chapter reviews and analyses the most appropriate and important research literature currently available;

4. The '*Recommendations for clinical practice*' offers suggestions for sound clinical practice based on the author's interpretation of the literature;

5. The '*Practice check*' enables professionals to examine their own practice and the principles and policies influencing their work;

6. Bibliographic sources are covered under *References* (to research) and *Suggestions for further reading*.

■ References

House of Commons Health Committee 1992 Report on the maternity services (Winterton Report). HMSO, London

Shepherd T 1990 Resourcing Project 2000 courses: the role of library and information services. Nursing Information Subgroup of the Library Association/RCN Library, London

■ Further reading on research

The titles listed below are suggested for those who wish to further their knowledge and understanding of the principles of research.

Cormack DFS (ed) 1991 The research process in nursing, 2nd ed. Blackwell Scientific Publications, Oxford

Distance Learning Centre Packages (1988–1992) Research awareness: a programme for nurses, midwives and health visitors, Units 1–13. South Bank Polytechnic, London

Field PA, Morse JM 1985 Nursing research: the application of qualitative approaches. Croom Helm, London

Hicks C 1990 Research and statistics: a practical introduction for nurses. Prentice Hall, Hemel Hempstead

Hockey L 1985 Nursing research – mistakes and misconceptions. Churchill Livingstone, Edinburgh

Chapter 1

Communication in Midwifery

Mavis Kirkham

When a midwife and a woman are together there is always communication, though the midwife will not always be seeking to give information. The midwife may communicate her busyness, her attention may be primarily focused on the monitor, the computer or the notes. The woman may receive a clear message of, 'I am concentrating, do not disturb', and act accordingly though the midwife is not aware that she is communicating.

Research shows that women want information about their condition and their care, and that good communication is highly valued. Good communication is very personal because it must be appropriate to the individuals involved. Research can give us guidelines and insights but care must be tailored to the individual.

Communication is also highly political because in the way we communicate we make a statement about the priorities we hold and where this woman fits into our priorities. Real communication is two way. Hospitals are not designed to foster two way communication in any depth. If we can achieve communication with women in our care which is really two way we enable women to tell their concerns and we listen. We must then reply appropriately to each individual woman. But knowledgeable women can make decisions and rock boats. If midwives choose not to respond to womens' search for information their choice may not be at a conscious level but it is not accidental. Communication is challenging, as are relationships, to which communication is fundamental.

■ **It is assumed that you are already aware of the following:**

- The complex communication skills you have developed through life in society;

- Communication systems within hospital hierarchies and their effect on patients and staff at various levels.

■ Making use of research to improve our communication skills

Communication cannot be described as just a part of midwifery care. 'To impart or exchange information, ideas or feelings' (Collins Dictionary) is fundamental to midwifery. Communication is the vehicle by which all else is learnt and relationships are built. Communication cannot be separated from other areas of care because care is built on and of communication. Cartwright's (1987) findings show this clearly: 'The main characteristics of the care mothers perceived as kind and understanding that have been identified are explanation and information and keeping pain and discomfort within their expectations...' Good care must involve sensitive communication. Good communication is concerned with the 'exchange of information, ideas or feelings' so that both parties understand more and have appropriate expectations. Just 'to impart' our instructions cannot be called good care.

In trying to improve communication, there are a number of different types of research which can be useful and there are different ways in which we can make use of that research.

□ What do women want?

Research asking women about their experience of the maternity services shows clearly a desire for intelligible, consistent information with which they can orientate themselves to their situation (Cartwright 1979; Kirke 1980; Oakley 1980). Green *et al* (1988), for instance, concluded 'The majority of women wanted to know as much as possible about what might happen in labour'. This desire for information must be seen in a larger context, for many studies (e.g. Cartwright 1964) show communication failure to be the patients' most commonly voiced criticism of health care in general.

There has been sufficient research into women's views of their care for conclusions to be drawn and practical suggestions made. Read and Garcia (1989) did this for antenatal screening:

> These studies show that, on average, the more information women
> receive, the less anxious they become ... Simple explanation and time
> spent on reassurance is well repaid: women report greater
> satisfaction with the whole procedure.

On non-routine antenatal tests Read and Garcia summarised the research into very practical suggestions:

> ... women wished to receive the report of results as quickly, and as
> personally as possible. They appreciate letters or telephone calls more
> than being left to assume that if not informed, all is well, but most
> prefer to be told in person.

The desire for information is similarly an important theme throughout women's experience of antenatal care (Macintyre 1982; Porter & Macintyre 1989), inpatient care (Perkins 1978; Kirkham 1989) and postnatal care in the community (Ball 1987, 1989). Martin (1990) has findings, which reflect many other studies, in showing communication to be central to women's understanding and appreciation of their care. 'At all stages of maternity care, the quality of communication between women and professional staff was a crucial determinant of satisfaction with care'.

All women may seek this information but whether or not they receive it is often related to social class, women of lower social class being likely to receive less information (Cartwright 1979). This 'Inverse Care Law' (Tudor Hart 1971) applies in maternity care and general medical care (Tudor Hart 1971; Arnold 1987; Jacoby 1988) and has long been known to apply to the giving of information (Pratt *et al* 1957). This may not be too surprising in the United Kingdom but it is found in some other settings. In an Australian study Shapiro and her colleagues (1983) concluded 'Lower social class patients desire more and obtain less information than their higher status counterparts'. So it appears likely that this problem is linked to care and the way it is delivered and not just to the British class system.

Another important factor influencing the information women receive is language. In a study of the views of linkworkers/interpreters in nine health districts, Hayes (1991) found that the majority did not think non-English speaking women were given as much information as English speaking women about their care in pregnancy, labour and childbirth. Without information even those non-English speakers lucky enough to have access to a link worker are unlikely to be able to make choices concerning their care.

□ **Expectations**

Research which asks questions of large numbers of women is built on the assumption that those women have clear views and are articulate in expressing them. This may not always be the case and here again women of lower social class are likely to lose out. In looking at 'What do women want? Asking consumers views', Perkins (1991) says:

> Part of the explanation for midwives' failure to identify some
> women's needs lies with the difficulty they may have in expressing
> them. Women may lack practice in identifying their own needs, lack
> confidence in expressing them or have no expectations that the
> service will be interested in them anyway.

She goes on to look at studies, such as that by Evans (1987), which identify examples of women who received clearly inadequate care and expressed only mild criticism, or none at all, when asked to assess their satisfaction with that care. We could conclude from this that women are satisfied whatever their care and seek very little from that care. Or we could conclude with Perkins (1991) that, 'It is always wise to assume that complaints or expressions of dissatisfaction should be taken seriously, they may well represent the tip of an iceberg'. We also need to remember women who cannot express their opinions in surveys because they are illiterate or cannot speak English or who, for whatever reason, do not respond to questionnaires. When reading research findings we need to bear in mind the possible 'iceberg' of non-respondents.

Beyond this we need to think about the nature of expectations and satisfaction. Our expectations are built from what we see as possible. Women are unlikely, particularly when experiencing unfamiliar organisations or the pain of labour, to have unrealistically high expectations. It may be argued that women are very realistic in their expectations of the maternity services and their realistically low expectations are usually satisfied. Such a view would accept that working class women may not receive care appropriate to their needs (Tudor Hart 1971) but still express a relatively low level of dissatisfaction with that care and the communication surrounding it (McIntosh 1989). Literature on postnatal depression (for example, Pitt 1968; McIntosh 1989) could lead us on to conclude that women need to be realistic in their expectations of our imperfect service for high expectations which are not met may be damaging.

If women's expectations are usually realistically low then it is of interest to look at research where women received care different from what is usual in their setting. Brooks (1990) found that when women can expect continuity of midwifery care their expectations and potential for satisfaction change accordingly. These women expected information and a high standard of communication based on a detailed knowledge of their situation because this was what they received from their community midwife. They expected to be so informed and to make choices based upon that information. If referred to hospital they found the communication in antenatal clinic very worrying. Also of interest are interviews where women were encouraged to look at the care they would ideally like from a midwife as distinct from the care they actually received (Kirkham 1987). When asking this in postnatal interviews with women whose labour I had observed, most stressed that their ideal midwife would 'explain' though many spoke kindly of their actual midwives who had not done so.

Studies where women speak about needs which they may not have articulated before involve the building of a trusting relationship with the researcher. Such studies are looking at a small number of women and cannot make wider generalisable statements. These qualitative studies therefore cannot tell us in general terms what we ought to do. They can give us insights into the care we give and how we can improve it. Such insights can shed light on the care we give to individuals, increase the repertoire of care we can offer and help us choose more sensitively the right care for each woman.

☐ Looking at communication: detachment and observation

Reading qualitative research can affect us in another useful way. The researcher must be simultaneously involved with the woman and sufficiently detached to analyse. The midwife who wishes to communicate well is in a similar position; she is highly observant of the woman in her care and of her own role with regard to that woman. Only with such awareness can she make full use of her experience and consciously improve her skills. So there are practical midwifery lessons to learn from research methods as well as research findings. This is particularly useful with regard to observation and interviewing skills.

If we adopt a 'researcher' attitude, where we are on the lookout for clues as to women's needs and better ways of explaining things around birth, we may find revelations in other places besides research reports. Books that have helped me in this respect include novels, poems and collections of birth stories (e.g. Sorel 1984).

Research that can help us in improving our communication skills is not confined to midwifery. Work on the use of language, such as Tannen's (1991) work on conversation between men and women, has implications that extend well beyond the workplace. 'When we think we are using language, our language is using us', is the thought provoking conclusion to a very readable chapter: 'Language keeps women in their place'.

Research on communication in other professional fields can also help us. See, for example, the work of Gask *et al* (1987, 1988) on training to improve communication in consultations between GPs and patients, and Crute *et al* (1989) on a communication skills course for student health visitors. The use of such techniques as open questions and clarifying comments are equally relevant in midwifery, as is learning not to interrupt clients. The teaching techniques would also be relevant to midwife teachers.

It is not just at work that we communicate. So efforts to improve our communication skills prove useful in many aspects of life which in turn feed back into our skills as midwives.

■ Looking at communication in its context

We usually accept our working situation as normal. We rarely seek to analyse the extent to which the institution or organisation in which we work modifies our actions and our views of ourselves, women in our care and our colleagues. Yet our setting is likely to have a profound effect on the professional self we present to women in our care (Goffman 1959).

Many problems in communication clearly stem from the way in which care is organised. Good communication is a two way process between equals. Much maternity care is conducted in circumstances where such equality is almost impossible to achieve – such as busy antenatal clinics where care is highly fragmented and many women have to be seen in a session. Where care is fragmented and notes are 'medical', it is difficult for a midwife to know what the woman already knows or wishes to know. Nor can communication in one visit be easily developed further in the future.

If all communication with women is a matter of starting from scratch, it is no wonder that communication is inadequate and mainly one way. When they are under such pressures, it is hardly surprising that midwives tend to explain more to women they feel are more likely to understand and too often give reassurancing noises rather than information. The relationships that have continuity in hospital are likely to be with staff rather than clients, and our wish to fit in socially will reinforce the hospital hierarchy.

Research on maternity care in hospital (Riley 1977; Kirkham 1987; Porter & Macintyre 1989) shows the medicalised nature of the setting and the position of women as passive work objects. The conveyor belt analogy is very striking. In this setting 'only "patients" who could prove themselves trustworthy or humble, that is, unlikely to be disruptive, were offered information which, if offered to others, might lead to inappropriate patient actions, and thus threaten the smooth flow of work through the ward' (Kirkham 1987). These midwives were not unkind, they had simply adapted to fit smoothly into their work setting which was medically dominated and hierarchical. This was demonstrated in the way in which midwives did not explain to mothers in the presence of doctors or senior midwives but as soon as the senior person left the room. The same study also produced the contrasting finding that the GP unit was the midwives' setting where the main person the midwife had to please was the mother. The woman in the GP unit had to cope with her labour and co-operate with her midwife much more actively than in the consultant unit as there was no epidural service. To achieve this midwives gave much more information and support and there were no senior staff to inhibit their information giving. In home births the home was the family's territory. There was no offstage professional area and the midwife was treated as a guest whose role was to respond appropriately to her hostess, answering questions and offering information. Thus roles are reversed, for the hospital patient seeks to please the staff whose territory she is on and she will rapidly cease to question if staff actions suggest that they are too busy to answer.

Continuity of care is clearly important here. Flint (1991) found that women in her 'Know your midwife scheme' were more likely to feel well prepared for labour, to have felt in control during labour and to have been satisfied with pain relief despite receiving less analgesia than the control group. They were also more likely to feel well prepared for childcare and able to discuss problems postnatally. Similarly, when comparing the views of women seeing few caregivers antenatally and those receiving a conventional regime, O'Brien and Smith (1981) found those with few caregivers were 'significantly more able to discuss things'. Much research still needs to be done on continuity of care for we cannot just assume that improved communication will follow. Currell (1990) studied the organisation of care and proposes a 'unity of care' where the individual woman and her family is the centre of the care which is 'focused' on her needs. This would certainly avoid situations where changes in organisation are assumed to improve care, such as creating teams of midwives which are far too large to offer continuity to any individual woman.

Written records are important in what they convey and who has access to them. Two experimental studies comparing woman-held obstetric records with conventional systems (Elbourne *et al* 1987; Lovell *et al* 1987) found that women who held their own records felt more in control of their antenatal care and more able to communicate effectively with staff. Clearly this was a move towards the equality that makes for good communication. A study of client held health visiting records (Jackson 1991) showed such equality transforming care and staff morale. Communication improved and insights were gained, such as when 'an Asian client wrote in her record in her own language... – what that meant for us was that we needed an interpreter – not her'. Such a situation is inconceivable in most hospital antenatal clinics where women so often feel 'You can't really ask' verbal questions (Kensington, Chelsea and Westminster CHC 1980; Porter & Macintyre 1989; Read & Garcia 1989).

Computerised records pose further problems in communication at all levels. The body language of an interview is totally transformed by the midwife entering information into a computer. The Deputy Health Service Ombudsman (quoted by Friend 1992) sees computerised records as problematic as they can encourage us to 'use pat standard phrases, encouraging a regimented approach'. Computers certainly solve the problem of making records legible but much needs to be done to make the language clear and accessible to women. Research needs to be done to help us grasp the opportunities offered by the 1990 Access to Health Records Act which prompts us to maintain written records which women can read on a basis of equality with staff.

Methven (1989) studied hospital antenatal booking interviews and found that, in laying the foundation for maternity records, 'midwives demonstrated very few devices for developing conversation or for probing in order to obtain salient facts'. She linked this finding to the context of the interview in observing 'that the style of questioning and interview technique were influenced primarily by pressure of time and workload, and secondly by poor role models when skills were being learnt'. Methven contrasted the traditional obstetric format booking interview with a nursing process format and demonstrated that the latter 'would enable a midwife to explore the woman's feelings and expectations which ... are relevant to the planning of her subsequent care'.

Research on information booklets for women also shows that much work needs to be done to overcome our history of using leaflets that are at‹

once patronising in the way they address women (Graham 1977) and heavily weighted with advertising. Efforts are currently being made to produce leaflets which can form a basis for real communication (Crawford 1992).

Defensive medicine is another important factor in the context of communication between midwives and mothers. The widespread medical fear of litigation can affect midwives too and the defensive attitudes that follow such fear can prevent midwives communicating with mothers as equals. Research shows that here again information is of crucial importance. 'Information and accountability are seen as central to the needs of medical accident victims' (Jones 1991). These concerns are also apparent in other countries and other areas of women's health (McGregor Vennell 1989). Jones (1991) speaks in words which are clearly applicable to our practice as midwives:

> What patients need when things have gone wrong is to know that they *have* gone wrong…, why things went wrong and to be given an apology. They need to know that other health professionals will be told that something has gone wrong, … and that everything possible will be done to put things right. Finally they need to know what action will be taken to ensure that similar accidents do not occur in the future.

Similarly Friend (1991) states, 'Studies show that in over 70% of incidents which progress to a lawsuit, patients would have been satisfied with someone saying, "I am sorry this happened"'. To achieve this, good communication must be the accepted practice when things are going right. Apology is then logical in the context of communication between equals as well as being the 'first rule of risk management' (Kent 1991). When defensive medicine is part of the context of our work it is a comfort to midwives to know that legal research shows that honesty is the best policy.

■ Learning from the research

If we are to improve our communication skills, then it is important to look at the basic principles involved in good practice before looking at midwifery care in its various parts.

Research suggests that midwives are skilled in clinical observation (McKay & Roberts 1990). Other pressures upon midwives, especially in hospital, often result in less attention being given to the observation of other cues from women in their care (Kirkham 1987; Porter & Macintyre 1989). Being aware of midwives' other priorities, women are hesitant to ask questions (Read & Garcia 1989) and this results in midwives lacking knowledge of women's specific needs and therefore being unable to tailor care to suit the individual.

If our meetings with women in our care are professionally controlled, women become patients and sink into the 'learned helplessness' (Seligman 1975) which is so destructive and depressing. Changes which are likely to improve communication are those which change the balance of power in favour of the woman. We need to let women speak in order to know their concerns and to improve our ability to listen to women's words and cues. Letting women speak may be a subtle skill to exercise with women who are unaccustomed to being heard.

☐ **Organisation of care**

If good communication follows from a relationship of equality between midwife and mother, then we must work for any changes in the organisation of care which are moves in that direction. Small teams of midwives providing continuity of care are likely to be a good way of fostering such equality (Flint 1991).

Changes which lessen medical pressures upon midwives are also likely to make their relationships with mothers more central to their concern; for instance midwives' beds in hospital, midwives' clinics and midwife/GP units.

If we can increase the amount of care women receive on their own territory, this is likely to help to change their status from patienthood to equality with staff. In the Newcastle Community Midwifery Care project, for instance, outcome was improved for a very vulnerable group of women. An intensive programme of home visiting improved relationships with mothers and 'improved women's confidence and understanding so that they were able to make informed use of the hospital services and this, in turn, improved their satisfaction with them' (Evans 1991).

☐ **Attitudes and skills**

As midwives we are likely to understand that women value good communication and to value it ourselves (Kirkham 1987). We already have high levels of skill in communication as women (Tannen 1991) and as midwives (McKay & Roberts 1990). It is likely to be helpful if we can raise our awareness of our own skills, as well as our limitations, before planning how these skills can be improved. Sometimes research can help us do this. McKay and Roberts' (1990) article 'Obstetrics by ear' is fascinating in showing midwives' skill in interpreting sounds made by women in labour. Honest feedback from trusted colleagues, self awareness study days and the habit of detached observation can all help us to increase our awareness of our existing level of skill in communication.

Working in small groups is usually the most fruitful way of both generating the confidence to work on our skills and improving our communication skills as midwives. We are fortunate in having some good learning materials to work from such as Eastcott and Farmer's (1989) package *Communication Skills for Midwifery and Other Health Care Professions*. Most inservice training departments would be happy to provide a facilitator for such a small group to meet regularly and enable each member to set herself appropriate plans to work on her skills in practice between meetings. If such educational support is not available it is possible for a group to work from distance learning materials (Bond 1991, or one of the many packs for nurses) or books (for example, Nelson-Jones 1986, or Scammell 1990). An individual can also do this but support and feedback help a lot.

In small group work to improve communication skills each midwife can choose to concentrate on an aspect she particularly wishes to work on. Issues here may be chosen as a result of experience or may be raised by research. Examples of areas raised by research are:

• Raising our awareness of womens' cues (Kirkham 1983, 1987);

• Communication during admission in labour (Garforth & Garcia 1987);

• Improving our skills in report giving (Hunt 1989);

• Improving our written notes (Methven 1989; Jackson 1991);

• Improving communication in antenatal classes (Murphy-Black & Faulkner 1990).

There is much scope for midwife teachers to create materials that can be used by small groups of midwives seeking to improve their skills. Much can be learnt from work on communication skills in other professions (Gask *et al* 1987, 1988; Crute *et al* 1989). Video can be a useful tool and would be one way of using Porter and Macintyre's (1989) recommendations:

> ... more attention should be devoted to ensuring that the care [women] are offered when they do attend [antenatal clinic] is beneficial, both clinically and psychologically. Although it may be distressing to the professionals involved, one mechanism for doing this is to show from direct observations, what is actually done and said in interactions with clients – which may be very different from what the professionals perceive themselves to be saying and doing.

A small and well facilitated group would be essential so that any distress resulting from such an exercise could be used constructively.

Women find it hard to ask questions of midwives and doctors unless they are specifically encouraged to do so (Read & Garcia 1989), as questions have been observed to be ignored or conversation blocked or deflected away from the point of enquiry (Kirkham 1987). This search for information may then be pursued by means of techniques which emphasise the woman's acceptance of her humble patient role, such as eavesdropping teaching of students and self-denigration (Kirkham 1987). Such techniques are successful to a certain extent, especially if contrasted with direct questions which may be unanswered or lead to midwives practising 'verbal asepsis' (Kitzinger 1978) – the conversational non-touch technique which avoids the woman's area of concern. Yet the very passivity of information-seeking techniques such as eavesdropping limits both their usefulness and the relevance of information gained for the individual woman. The humble eavesdropper cannot ask for explanations.

Knowing the problems with regard to asking questions can provide us with a way to monitor our efforts to improve our skills as midwives. If we offer information and seek questions, women see that we wish to communicate and are likely to ask questions because we have shown this to be our aim. Similarly if we answer questions immediately and clearly, women are likely to feel free to ask further because our behaviour shows that we see this woman's knowledge and understanding to be important. As we try to develop ways of improving our communication skills, women's questions and responses can show whether we are succeeding. As Currell (1990) stated, 'Women report satisfaction with antenatal care where they feel they have been given reassurance and their questions have been answered'. This is an important and complex issue from which we can learn much: Green *et al* (1988) concluded 'Psychological outcomes, particularly satisfaction and emotional wellbeing are related to the answers women gave antenatally to questions about information and communication with staff'.

Encouraging and monitoring questions can be a useful approach throughout midwifery care. It can, for instance, be useful in antenatal classes in moving the balance of the class from the midwife giving information to parents discussing their concerns. This would help to meet the need for antenatal education tailored to individuals' requirements – a need revealed by research in many countries (Rautava *et al* 1990). There may also be times, for instance when labour is very painful, when another approach, such as a gentle running commentary, enables the woman to be informed but only respond when she wishes (Kirkham 1987).

Reading research can help us raise our self-awareness and highlight specific areas where we may work on our communication skills. Reassurance has been one of these areas for me. In observing communication in labour (Kirkham 1987, 1989), I heard midwives 'reassuring' women with phrases which contained no information such as, 'We [staff] will worry about that' or 'You're in the right place'. Often the reassurance consisted of a command to the woman 'not to worry'. Women are very likely to comply with their midwife's wishes and if the worry is not raised again this may lead the midwife to assume that her reassurance was effective. This is unlikely to be true. The very fact that women are so eager to please the midwife means that when she says 'Don't worry' she effectively says 'Shut up'. Hays and Larson (1963) state this in more theoretical terms:

> attempting to dispel the patient's anxiety by implying that there is not sufficient reason for it to exist is to completely devalue the patient's own feelings ... There is absolutely no justification for trying to reassure, unless you are able to document what you say.

Teasdale (1989) usefully distinguishes between reassurance as a 'purposeful attempt to restore confidence' and reassurance as an 'optimistic assertion'. We can use this distinction to plan ways of restoring women's confidence. It also helps us beware of using phrases aimed at cheering ourselves in our conversation with patients. Phrases such as 'That's not bad is it?' or 'It's never as bad as you think it is' from the midwife rob the woman of words and certainly do not aid communication. Similarly we should not justify procedures as being of immediate help to the woman unless we ensure that this is so (Kirkham 1987, 1989). Otherwise we reassure ourselves by confusing the needs of our organisation with the felt needs of individual women. One thing that convinces me of the practical use of research is the way midwives I do not know quite often greet me with the words, 'Oh, you're the person who stopped me saying "don't worry".' The pressures on us often make us want to say 'don't worry'. But if the words slip out we can at least follow them with 'because ...'.

Sometimes there are reasons to worry and there we can help women to be prepared. Women want to be prepared in this sense (Green *et al* 1988) and we have long acknowledged this fundamental need by providing antenatal classes. There is much nursing literature on the benefits of such preparation before surgery for instance (Tarasuk *et al* 1965; Hayward 1975; Boore 1978). Midwives often appear afraid that the patient may worry but the psychological literature (Janis 1968) suggests that the preparatory 'work of worrying' improves the individual's psychological and physiological coping mechanisms. If this work is to be done it falls to the midwife to help by providing information and support.

Communication with doctors is another area where we need to increase our self awareness for the sake of women in our care. Twenty-five years ago Stein described 'the doctor-nurse game':

> The object of the game is as follows: the nurse is to be bold, have initiative and be responsible for making significant recommendations, while at the same time she must appear passive. This must be done in such a manner so as to make her recommendations appear to be initiated by the physician. (Stein 1967)

This is also played as the doctor-midwife game by midwives who are at the same time maintaining the order of the ward as expected by senior medical staff and taking a major part in the training and socialisation of junior medical staff (Kirkham 1987). Stein (1990) finds the doctor-nurse game is changing due to many factors including improved nurse education, 'that force within the human condition that moves us from dependence towards autonomy and mutual interdependence' and the development of the 'stubborn rebel' within the nursing profession. Such changes could equally be cited in midwifery but we lack the research and possibly the self awareness of nurses in this area.

The doctor-nurse game is a devious and limited way of communicating. It reinforces hierarchical relationships and, when played in the presence of women in our care, highlights their position at the bottom of the hierarchy and our subservient role as midwives. Increasing our self awareness and skills in communication with doctors is likely to have a positive effect on communication far beyond the immediate encounter.

Conversation between doctors and midwives often highlights issues in conversation between men and women where the male speaker assumes the power to interrupt and redirect conversation (Spender 1980). There are striking parallels between the humble techniques that women use with midwives and midwives in turn use with doctors to gain information (Kirkham 1987). Such humility is tragic, not least because it is inefficient. With self awareness and planning, attitudes and relationships can change (Jackson 1991).

Changes in attitudes and development of skills such as those described above would have a profound effect upon the care we give and the women and colleagues we work with. Such changes, in turn, can lead to changes in organisational structures. Thus a positive spiral of change can be created of which we are all part.

For us to bring about change, either in ourselves or in structures, we need support. Such support must be strengthening if it is to be useful. We are scarcely likely to be able to empower women if we feel powerless ourselves. Research in other helping professions shows the need and potential use of such support (Hawkins & Shohet 1989) and research on this matter is much needed in midwifery. Support can come from supervision, in the sense in which that word is used by counsellors to mean a system of support from respected colleagues with whom we can analyse our practice and learn from it in safety. Support may also come from small groups of colleagues, possibly arising from the sort of educational exercise suggested above, or in the form of midwives' meetings within a team or workplace set up for this purpose. Or support may be gained from a local branch of a midwives' organisation or one of the many organisations of women who share with us the aim of improving the maternity services.

■ Recommendations for clinical practice in the light of currently available evidence

1. Women want to be prepared for the experiences of the childbearing year. It should, therefore, be an important part of our work as midwives to help women and families gain the information and make the decisions which enable each individual to cope best.

2. Midwives should offer information to women and not wait to be asked. Questions should be encouraged and answered honestly.

3. Women should carry their own maternity records and understand them with their midwives' help.

4. Good communication is two way and likely to be aided by relationships of equality. We must, therefore, aim to give care in such a way that women and midwives work in equal partnership. Continuity of care may well provide a good setting for such a partnership. Much may also be achieved by giving more care on the woman's own territory or changing the organisation of care so that midwives are better able to listen to women.

5. Similarly, we should avoid ways of communicating with colleagues or clients which reinforce power differences – such as playing the 'doctor-nurse game' or giving unsubstantiated 'reassurance' to women.

6. Midwives have high levels of skill in clinical observation. Self-awareness is fundamental to developing these skills further to improve communication. Self-awareness and specific communication skills can be developed most easily by work in small groups in a safe setting.

7. Progress in communication is likely to proceed best where midwives have a good system of personal support and supervision.

■ Practice check

- What strategies have you found successful in helping women to ask questions and voice their concerns?

- What do you do non-verbally that puts women at ease and improves communication?

- What facilities do you have to aid communication with women who do not speak English? Can you do anything to improve this?

- When teaching a student in the presence of a woman in your care, do you specifically include that woman in the teaching? How does that affect the interaction? What may the student and the woman assume from that about your priorities?

- How often do you say 'Don't worry' to women in your care? Is this constructive? If you find yourself saying 'Don't worry' try to follow it with 'because...' Note the woman's response.

- When you learn a new piece of information about a woman, however small, do you tell her? What does your action convey to her?

- How are test results given to women in your antenatal clinic? Could this be done better?

- Monitor the time you speak and the time parents speak in your next antenatal class. Would it be useful to change this? If so how?

- Try giving women in your care a gentle running commentary on your actions so as to increase their peace of mind and potential for choice. Note the women's response.

- What have you done this week to counteract the Inverse Care Law? And what have you done to promote continuity of care?

- Does your in-service training department run courses for midwives to improve their skills in communication, counselling and assertiveness? If not, have you asked for them?

- Where do you get your support as a midwife? Could you improve your support base?

■ References

Arnold M 1987 The cycle of maternal deprivation. Midwife, Health Visitor and Community Nurse 23 (12): 539–42

Ball J A 1987 Reactions to motherhood: The roll of postnatal care. Cambridge University Press, Cambridge

Ball J A 1989 Postnatal care and adjustment to motherhood. In Robinson S, and Thomson AM (eds) Midwives, research and childbirth, Vol 1. Chapman and Hall, London

Bond M 1991 Assertiveness for midwives. Distance Learning Centre, South Bank Polytechnic, London

Boore J R P 1978 Prescription for recovery. RCN, London

Brooks F 1990 Alternative to the medical model of childbirth: a qualitative study of user-centred maternity care. Unpublished PhD thesis, University of Sheffield

Cartwright A 1964 Human relations and hospital care. Routledge and Kegan Paul, London

Cartwright A 1979 The dignity of labour: a study of childbirth and induction. Tavistock Publications, London

Cartwright A 1987 Who are maternity services kind to? What is 'kindness'? Midwife, Health Visitor and Community Nurse   23 (1): 21–4

Crawford D 1992 Putting parents in the picture. Nursing Times   88 (2): 41–2

Crute V C, Hargie O D W, Ellis R A F 1989 An evaluation of a communication skills course for health visitor students. Journal of Advanced Nursing   14: 546–52

Currell R 1990 The organisation of midwifery care. In Alexander J, Levy V, Roch S (eds) Antenatal care: a research-based approach (Midwifery Practice, Vol 1). Macmillan, Basingstoke

Eastcott D, Farmer B 1989 Communication skills for midwifery and other health care professions: learning materials. West Midlands Health Authority and Birmingham Polytechnic Learning Methods Unit, Birmingham

Elbourne D, Richardson M, Chalmers I, Waterhouse I, Holt E 1987 The Newbury Maternity Care Study: a randomised controlled trial to evaluate a policy of women holding their own maternity records. British Journal of Obstetrics and Gynaecology   94: 612–19

Evans F B 1987 The Newcastle Community Midwifery Care Project: an evaluation report. Newcastle Health Authority Community Health Unit, Newcastle

Evans F B 1991 The Newcastle Community Midwifery Care Project: The evaluation of the project. In Robinson S, Thomson A M Midwives, research and childbirth, Vol 2. Chapman and Hall, London

Flint C 1991 Continuity of care provided by a team of midwives – the Know Your Midwife Scheme. In Robinson S, Thomson A M Midwives, research and childbirth, Vol 2. Chapman and Hall, London

Flint C, Poulengeris P 1987 The 'Know your midwife' report. Privately printed; available from 49 Peckarmans Wood, Sydenham Hill, London SE26 6RZ

Friend B 1991 Cutting the risks. Nursing Times   87 (17): 44–5

Friend B 1992 Record recovery. Nursing Times   88 (2): 34–5

Garforth S, Garcia J 1987 Admitting – a weakness or a strength? Routine admission of a woman in labour. Midwifery   3 (1): 10–24

Gask L, Goldberg D, Lesser A L, Millar T 1988 Improving the psychiatric skills of the general practice trainee: an evaluation of a group training course. Medical Education   22: 132–8

Gask L, McGrath G, Goldberg D, Millar T 1987 Improving the psychiatric skills of established general practitioners: evaluation of group teaching. Medical Education   21: 362–8

Goffman E 1959 The presentation of self in everyday life. Penguin, Harmondsworth

Goffman E 1961 Asylums: Essays on the social situation of mental patients and other inmates. Penguin, Harmondsworth

Graham H 1977 Images of pregnancy in ante-natal literature. In Dingwall R, Heath C, Reid M, Stacey M Health care and health knowledge. Croom Helm, London

Green J M, Coupland V A, Kitzinger JV 1988 Great expectations: a prospective study of women's expectations and experiences of childbirth. Child Care and Development Group, University of Cambridge

Hawkins P, Shohet R 1989 Supervision and the helping professions. Open University Press, Milton Keynes

Hayes L 1991 Communication in the maternity services. Maternity Action 50, (July/August): 6–7

Hays J, Larson K H 1963 Interacting with patients. Macmillan Inc, New York

Hayward J 1975 Information – A prescription against pain, RCN, London

Hunt S 1989 The labour ward – A midwife's castle? Research and the Midwife Conference Proceedings (Available from the University of Manchester, Department of Nursing Studies)

Jackson C 1991 Power to the parent. Health Visitor 64 (10): 340–342

Jacoby A 1988 Mothers' views about information and advice in pregnancy and childbirth: Findings from a national study. Midwifery 4: 103–110

Janis I L 1968 When fear is healthy. Psychology Today 1: 46–9; 60–61

Jones M L 1991 The no-fault compensation debate. Association of Personal Injury Lawyers, Proceedings of the Spring Meeting May 1

Kent P 1991 Letter to the Editor. Health Service Journal 101 (5244): 10

Kensington, Chelsea and Westminster (South) Community Health Council 1980 Maybe I didn't ask: A report on the experience of women having their babies in Westminster Hospital. Kensington, Chelsea and Westminster CHC, London

Kirke P N 1980 Mothers' views of obstetric care. British Journal of Obstetrics and Gynaecology 87: 1029–33

Kirkham M J 1983 Labouring in the dark: Limitations on the giving of information to enable patients to orientate themselves to the likely events and timescale of labour. In Wilson-Barnett J (ed) Nursing research: Ten studies in patient care. John Wiley, Chichester

Kirkham M J 1987 Basic supportive care in labour: Interaction with and around labouring women. Unpublished PhD thesis, University of Manchester

Kirkham M J 1989 Midwives and information-giving during labour. In Robinson S, Thomson A M (eds) Midwives, research and childbirth, Vol 1. Chapman and Hall, London

Kitzinger S. 1978 Pain in childbirth. Journal of Medical Ethics 4 (Jan): 119–21

Lovell A, Zander L I, James C E, Foot S, Swan A V, Reynolds A 1987 The St Thomas's Maternity Case Notes Study: A randomised controlled trial to assess the effects of giving expectant mothers their own maternity case notes. Paediatric and Perinatal Epidemiology 1: 57–66

McGregor Vennell 1989 Medical misfortune in a no fault society. In Mann R D, Havard J (eds) No fault compensation in medicine. Joint Meeting of the Royal Society of Medicine and the British Medical Association, RSM, London

McIntosh J 1988 Women's views of communication during labour and delivery. Midwifery 4: 166–70

McIntosh J 1989 Models of childbirth and social class: a study of 80 working class primigravidae. In Robinson S, Thomson A M Midwives, research and childbirth, Vol 1. Chapman and Hall, London

McKay S, Roberts J 1990 Obstetrics by ear: maternal and caregiver perceptions of the meaning of maternal sounds during second stage labor. Journal of Nurse–Midwifery 35 (5): 266–73

Macintyre S 1982 Communications between pregnant women and their medical and midwifery attendants. Midwives Chronicle 95 (1138): 387–94

Martin C 1990 How do you count maternal satisfaction? A user-commissioned survey of maternity services. In Roberts H (ed) Women's health counts. Routledge, London

Methven R 1989 Recording an obstetric history or relating to a pregnant woman? A study of the antenatal booking interview. In Robinson S, Thomson A M (eds) Midwives, research and childbirth, Vol 1. Chapman and Hall, London

Murphy-Black T, Faulkner A 1990 Antenatal education. In Murphy-Black T, Faulkner A (eds) Excellence in nursing, the research route: Midwifery. Scutari Press, London

Nelson-Jones R 1986 Human relationship skills: training and self-help. Cassell, London

Oakley A 1980 Women confined: towards a sociology of childbirth. Martin Robertson, Oxford

O'Brien M, Smith C 1981 Women's views and experiences of antenatal care. Practitioner 25: 123–5

Perkins E R 1978 Having a baby: an educational experience? Leverhulme Health Education Project Occasional Paper No 6, University of Nottingham

Perkins E R 1991 What do women want? Asking consumers' views. Mabel Liddiard Memorial Lecture. Midwives Chronicle 104 (1247): 347–54

Pitt B 1968 Atypical depression following childbirth. British Journal of Psychiatry 114: 1325–35

Porter M, Macintyre S 1989 Psychosocial effectiveness of antenatal and postnatal care. In Robinson S, Thomson AM (eds) Midwives, research and childbirth, Vol 1. Chapman and Hall, London

Pratt L, Seligman A, Reader G 1957 Physicians' views of the level of medical information among patients. American Journal of Public Health 47: 1277–83

Rautava P, Erkkola R, Sillanpaa M 1990 The Finnish family competence study: new directions are necessary in antenatal education. Health Education Research 5 (3): 353–9

Read M, Garcia J 1989 Women's views of care during pregnancy and childbirth. In Enkin M W, Keirse M J N C, Chalmers I (eds) Effective care in pregnancy and childbirth: 131–42. Oxford University Press, Oxford

Riley E M D 1977 What do women want? The question of choice in the conduct of labour. In Chard T, Richards M (eds) Benefits and hazards of the new obstetrics. Heinemann/Spastics International Medical Publications, London

Scammell B 1990 Communication skills. Macmillan, Basingstoke, London

Seligman M E P 1975 Helplessness: On depression, development and death. Friedman, San Francisco

Shapiro M C, Najman J M, Chang A, Keeping J D, Morrison J, Western J S 1983 Information control and the exercise of power in the obstetrical encounter. Social Science and Medicine 17 (3): 139–46

Sorel N C 1984 Ever since Eve: Personal reflections on childbirth. Michael Joseph, London

Spender D 1980 Man made language. Routledge and Kegan Paul, London

Stein L 1967 The doctor-nurse game. Archives of General Psychiatry 16: 6698–703

Stein L, Watts D, Howell T 1990 The doctor-nurse game revisited. New England Journal of Medicine 332 (8): 546–9

Tannen D 1991 You just don't understand: Women and men in conversation. Virago, London

Tarasuk M B, Rhymes J A, Leonard R C 1965 An experimental test of the importance of communication skills for effective nursing. In Skipper J K, Leonard RC (eds) Social interaction and patient care. J B Lippincott, Philadelphia

Teasdale K 1989 The concept of reassurance in nursing. Journal of Advanced Nursing 14: 444–50

Tudor Hart J 1971 The Inverse Care Law. The Lancet VI: 405

■ Suggested further reading

Eastcott D, Farmer B 1989 Communication skills for midwifery and other healthcare professions: Learning materials. West Midlands Health Authority and Birmingham Polytechnic Learning Methods Unit, Birmingham

Henley N M 1977 Body politics: Power, sex and nonverbal communication. Touchstone, Simon and Schuster, New York

Read M, Garcia J 1989 Women's views of care during pregnancy and childbirth. In Enkin M W, Keirse M J N C, Chalmers I (eds) Effective care in pregnancy and childbirth: 131–42. Oxford University Press

Tannen D 1991 You just don't understand: Women and men in conversation. Virago, London

Chapter 2

Iron and vitamin supplementation during pregnancy

Elsa Montgomery

All midwives, in the course of their practice, encounter women who are on iron and vitamin supplements. In the case of iron, a doctor will usually have prescribed treatment, whereas vitamins may well have been bought over the counter. In either case, the real indication for such treatment is unclear.

Dietary supplementation during pregnancy has been advocated in this country since around the time of the Second World War, when concern about endemic maternal anaemia prompted routine iron prophylaxis. Such widespread prescription of vitamins has not yet occurred, but the use of vitamin tablets is nevertheless encouraged by their free availability to pregnant women on income support.

The need for a blanket approach to iron prophylaxis is now questioned, but there is controversy over the correct interpretation of research evidence. Studies on either the necessity for, or the prevalence of general vitamin supplementation in pregnancy are few. However, the potential for both benefit and hazard in the use of vitamins has recently been brought to public attention with the publication of the Medical Research Council study on prevention of neural tube defects (MRC Vitamin Study Research Group 1991) and by warnings from the Department of Health regarding high doses of vitamin A (DoH 1990).

This chapter discusses some of the relevant research into iron and vitamins to assist midwives in deciding what advice they should offer women about supplementation.

■ **It is assumed that you are already aware of the following:**

- Changes occurring in the blood during pregnancy;
- The meaning of basic haematological indices;

- Foods in which iron and vitamins are found;
- The functions of iron and vitamins.

■ Reasons for supplementation

Pregnant women are usually assumed to be in need of dietary supplements due to fetal demands on their supplies. As such they are regarded as a high risk group for deficiency (Truswell 1990); however, the evidence is equivocal. Most authorities seem to agree that there is no need for an increased intake of vitamins in a well nourished community (Drug and Therapeutics Bulletin 1984; Hytten 1990). The Panel on Dietary Reference Values of the Committee of Medical Aspects of Food Policy (1991) does not give pregnancy increments for most nutrients, as they believe that any extra demands should be met by normal adaptation, increased efficiency of utilisation, or from stores of the nutrient. Notwithstanding this, they still endorse the ready availability of vitamin supplements for pregnant and lactating women in case of inadequate stores.

In their study of the extent and determinants of vitamin supplementation in early pregnancy, Best *et al* (1989) discovered confusion over how appropriate such supplementation is thought to be. The 246 women who completed their questionnaire were recruited at antenatal clinics in one hospital. Women were more likely to receive advice from friends and relatives than from health professionals. Twenty three per cent of women took supplements (as determined by interview; frequency as determined by notes was only 8 per cent). Slightly more of these bought them over the counter than had them prescribed. Of those who gave details about the advice they received, fourteen women were advised in favour of supplementation and seven against. It was not possible to identify criteria for advising supplementation and there was no obvious pattern for regimens suggested. Those who advised against supplements did so on the grounds that they are unnecessary if a balanced diet is followed.

In the study of antenatal vitamin and iron supplementation in Glasgow by Bennett and McIlwaine (1985), 35 per cent of women were taking vitamins. In contrast to the results of Best *et al*, most (52 out of 66) were doing so on the advice of a medical practitioner. All but one of the 158 women were taking iron. Whilst most knew that this was related to blood, haemoglobin and anaemia, knowledge of reasons for vitamin supplementation was much less specific and only 32 per cent recalled learning anything from the prescriber. This does not necessarily imply that information was not given (indeed only 43 per cent of those taking iron reported the prescriber as a source of information) but it is worth noting, given the confusion found by Best *et al*.

A conspicuous lack of physiological data on the nutritional needs of pregnant women is described by Hytten (1990), who also notes a 'wealth of strongly held opinions' (page 95). Most pregnant women have iron and vitamin levels that are lower than those of non-pregnant women. The problem lies in deciding whether this is physiological or pathological (Hemminki & Starfield 1978). Koller (1982) states that 'the physiological parameters of pregnancy often resemble pathology in the non-pregnant state' (page 649) and Swinhoe *et al* (1989) note the difficulty in objective assessment of results which is consequent upon this.

■ Iron levels in pregnant women

The physiology and pathology debate has been widely studied in connection with iron supplementation.

□ Haemodilution

Haemodilution, which occurs progressively up to about 32 weeks of pregnancy, results in an apparent drop in iron levels as the proportional increase in plasma is greater than that in red blood cells (Hytten & Leitch 1971). It is known that oral iron therapy can prevent or at least modify this 'physiological anaemia'. Hytten (1985) estimates that the red blood cell mass increases by about 250 ml in non-supplemented women and by 400–450 ml in those taking iron. This could be suggestive of deficiency, the classical test for which is 'cure by replacement' (Hytten & Leitch 1971: page 37).

Some authors are thus concerned about iron levels and argue in favour of supplementation to ensure that fetal requirements are met (Fenton *et al* 1977) and to enable mothers to withstand any perinatal haemorrhage (Kelly *et al* 1977). Others affirm haemodilution as an important adaptation to pregnancy (Chesley 1972; Hytten 1985). Hytten (1985) suggests there is no reason to suppose the 250 ml increase in red blood cell volume in non supplemented women is inadequate. The oxygen carrying capacity of the blood is the important factor rather than iron levels *per se*. As the difference between arterial and venous oxygen concentrations is less in pregnant than in non-pregnant women, the oxygen-carrying capacity would appear to be adequate. Whereas the number of red blood cells are governed by the need to transport oxygen, plasma volume changes in relation to the need to fill the vascular space and maintain blood pressure. Chesley (1972) maintains that in pregnant women with a good diet, low haemoglobin usually points to a large plasma volume rather than deficiency in erythrocytes. This volume expansion serves to fill the increased vasculature of the pregnant uterus, allows dissipation of heat and provides reserves against pooling of blood in the lower extremities when supine. Furthermore, it reduces the viscosity of the blood causing a decreased resistance to flow and lowering the cardiac force required to propel blood round the body. Both Chesley (1972) and Hytten and Leitch (1971) cite studies which suggest that lack of haemodilution represents poor adaptation to pregnancy, leading to increased risk of pre-eclampsia in mothers and greater risk of abortion, stillbirth and low birthweight amongst babies. However, it is known that low levels of haemoglobin are also associated with low birthweight, preterm delivery and high perinatal mortality rates (Hemminki & Starfield 1978).

☐ **Measuring anaemia**

Whether or not low haemoglobin levels represent deficiency in pregnant women is obviously an important question to be answered. Whilst there is a physiological explanation for apparently low haemoglobin, the fact that its concentration can nevertheless be improved by supplements could equally indicate deficiency. Because of the changes described above, however, arbitrary levels of haemoglobin or red cell concentration are not useful parameters in pregnancy. For Hytten and Leitch (1971) the crucial information needed is about iron stores. They postulate that the falling concentration of iron could not be attributed to deficiency where there were demonstrable stores of unused iron.

Since they wrote that, it has become possible to determine iron stores by measuring serum ferritin. Fenton *et al* (1977) studied the iron stores of 154 women who attended the antenatal clinic within the first 14 weeks of pregnancy. The sample was divided into two groups according to the day on which they attended clinic. The first received prophylactic ferrous sulphate whilst the second did not receive supplements unless their haemoglobin fell below 11 g/dl, which it did in 42 (58 per cent) of the 72 women in the latter group. At term the haemoglobin concentration and mean corpuscular volume were basically unchanged in both groups. Transferrin saturation was lower in both groups than at booking and especially in untreated women. Serum iron had significantly declined only in those who were not given supplements. Serum ferritin levels fell in both groups. In the untreated women this occurred during the first 32 weeks of pregnancy, then levelled. When supplements were given a similar but less marked decline was seen until week 28 (see Tables 2.1 and 2.2 overleaf).

Twenty five of the women, taken from both groups, also had serum ferritin measured five to eight weeks after delivery. None of them had been supplemented in the puerperium, yet all showed serum ferritin concentrations not significantly different from those at booking. Forty one of the untreated women had stores at deficient levels at term even though their initial measurements were indistinguishable from other women. Levels of cord ferritin from the babies of these women were significantly reduced and Fenton *et al* found no evidence that the fetus has any priority over the

Table 2.1 Mean values for parameters of haematological and iron status at the week 10–14 of pregnancy. (Reproduced from Fenton *et al* 1977: 146, by kind permission of Blackwell Scientific Publications Ltd)

Patients	Hb (g/dl)	MCV (fl)	Serum iron (μmol/l)	Transferrin saturation (%)	Serum ferritin (μg/l)
Not treated (30)	12.9	88	23	36	96
Treated for anaemia (42)	12.3	86	21	31	71
Treated prophylactically (82)	12.5	86	22	33	67

Table 2.2 Mean values for parameters of haematological and iron status at term. (Reproduced from Fenton *et al* 1977: 146, by kind permission of Blackwell Scientific Publications Ltd)

Patients	Hb (g/dl)	MCV (fl)	Serum iron (μmol/l)	Transferrin saturation (%)	Serum ferritin (μg/l)
Not treated (30)	12.0	86	14	13	13
Treated for anaemia (42)	12.0	87	24	25	29
Treated prophylactically (82)	12.5	90	25	27	41

mother in its need for iron (this is in conflict with a later study which is discussed below). The authors conclude that during pregnancy the demand for iron far outstrips supply and there is a rapid decline in iron stores irrespective of whether supplements are taken, albeit less marked if they are. They believe that this increased demand must be due to a marked increase in erythropoietic activity occurring before the second trimester as fetal demands are not significant until much later in pregnancy. Thus only minimal stores remain by the time fetal requirements are greatest.

Kelly *et al* (1977) also report a significant decrease in plasma ferritin levels during the second half of pregnancy. They compared pregnant women, all of whom were receiving iron supplements, with a control group of non-pregnant women. Although there was little difference in plasma ferritin levels between the two groups before 25 weeks gestation and six days after delivery, there were highly significant differences at term. The reduction in iron stores as measured by plasma ferritin, once again occurred despite iron supplementation, albeit later in pregnancy than in the study by Fenton and colleagues. Kelly *et al* postulate that their research shows insufficient iron stores to meet the demands of pregnancy. Even with iron therapy they consider many women might not be able to respond to perinatal haemorrhage and recommend that iron supplementation be continued to maintain minimal stores.

Foulkes and Goldie (1982), in their study on the use of serum ferritin to assess the need for iron supplements in pregnancy, subdivided their two main groups of supplemented and non-supplemented women according to serum ferritin levels at booking. As in the study by Fenton *et al* (1977) if the non supplemented women became anaemic (in this case defined as a haemoglobin of less than 10.5 g/dl) they commenced oral iron therapy. Their final sample numbered 501 women. Overall 59 women developed haemoglobin levels of less than 10.5 g/dl before delivery.' Forty seven of these were in the 'unsupplemented' group – a much smaller proportion requiring treatment than in the study by Fenton *et al* (approximately 19 per cent as opposed to 58 per cent). In broad agreement with the other studies discussed, there was a marked fall in serum ferritin concentration in both groups by 28 weeks, the decline being greater in those not receiving supplements. In this latter group, levels continued to fall to 36 weeks. Those on iron maintained levels above 10 microgram/l. By the second day post partum, serum ferritin levels were two to three times those at 36 weeks. Forty one (87 per cent) of the unsupplemented women who became anaemic during the trial had serum ferritin levels of less than 50 microgram/l. Iron supplements did not alter the incidence of anaemia in those women with booking ferritin levels greater than 50 microgram/l and in those with booking ferritin levels over 80 microgram/l there was no difference in haematological variables irrespective of supplementation. These results lead Foulkes and Goldie to assert that serum ferritin may be usefully employed as a screen at booking and that those women with serum ferritin of less than 50 microgram/l should receive iron supplements.

Unlike Fenton *et al* (1977), Foulkes and Goldie found no difference in mean cord blood serum ferritin whether or not supplements were taken and they believe that fetal iron status is independent of maternal stores. Indeed, Fenton *et al* would appear to be in a minority with their findings that the fetus has no priority over the mother in its need for iron. The British Medical Journal (1978) asserts that maternal iron deficiency does not lead to low fetal levels and Bentley (1985) suggests that cord serum ferritin may be five times that of the mother.

□ **Utilisation of iron during pregnancy**

According to Svanberg (1975), daily iron requirement increases tenfold during pregnancy. This can either be covered by increased absorption or by mobilisation from stores. If these two sources are insufficient, deficiency will result in the absence of supplements. Absorption of iron is related to tissue iron stores and the rate of erythropoiesis. In early pregnancy, as described above, the red cell mass expands and iron stores are depleted. Absorption of iron at this stage is lower than in non-pregnant women and only increases later in the pregnancy (when fetal requirements are greater). This is true even in women receiving doses of supplements big enough to prevent depleted stores (Svanberg 1975).

☐   The significance of haemoglobin levels

At what level it becomes appropriate to boost haemoglobin with supplements remains an unanswered question. Foulkes and Goldie (1982) recognise the difficulties in separating pathological processes from physiological changes due to pregnancy alone. They note both the difficulties in defining anaemia in pregnancy and the variation in what is accepted as the lower limit of normal. According to Hytten and Leitch (1971), normality in pregnancy cannot be judged by reference to non-pregnant standards. Therein lies the biggest problem; for no one seems to know what is normal for the pregnant population. Studies performed either involve routine use of supplements or intervention with iron therapy when arbitrary haemoglobin levels are reached.

Concern has rightly focused on the association between low haemoglobin and high perinatal mortality, low birthweight and increased incidence of preterm births. It has been assumed that high haemoglobin would lead to a better outcome for both mother and baby. The work of Koller *et al* (1980), however, suggests that high haemoglobin levels (defined by the authors as two standard deviations above the mean value of normal distribution) during pregnancy may indicate a fetus at risk. They observed a link between high haemoglobin and both growth retardation and intrauterine death of unknown cause. Murphy *et al* (1986) studied the relationship between haemoglobin concentration at booking and subsequent outcome in 54 382 singleton pregnancies from the Cardiff Births Survey. They arranged haemoglobin values into three groups; low (<10.4 g/dl), intermediate (10.4–13.2 g/dl) and high (13.3 g/dl and above). Those with lower levels tended to have an excess of factors associated with being disadvantaged (such as low socioeconomic group, extremes of maternal age, smoking) – a point also raised by Hemminki and Starfield (1978). Maternal characteristics were similar in the other two groups. Looking at the variables of preterm births, low birthweight and perinatal deaths, they discovered a 'U-shaped' distribution. Women with high haemoglobin levels were as likely to have problems as those with low levels. They also found a clear association between high haemoglobin and hypertension and pre-eclampsia. While poor outcomes amongst those with low haemoglobin could be partly attributed to epidemiological factors, no such explanation could be proffered for those with high haemoglobin. The authors suggest that some failure in plasma expansion might be the cause. Both Koller *et al* and Murphy *et al* caution against routine iron prophylaxis.

■ The use of vitamins

As discussed earlier, routine vitamin supplements are not generally recommended and, unlike iron, widespread prescription has not occurred. There is, however, concern about inappropriate self-medication. Truswell (1990) comments on the general public's belief in vitamins (such as vitamin C to treat colds). While he sees no particular harm in supplementation, he sees no benefit either and warns of potential overdose or toxic effects. Best and colleagues (1989) express concern about the likelihood of restrictions on NHS prescriptions leading to more self-medication, and are particularly worried about the availability of high dose preparations in health food shops. How reasonable their concerns are is unclear. Bennett and McIlwaine (1985) found that most women taking vitamins had them prescribed by medical practitioners. More than half of the sample studied by Best *et al* (1989) bought 'over the counter' preparations, but only three women obtained them from health food shops. However, neither study was large scale (158 women and 246 women respectively) and the former involved women from a deprived area. A broader investigation might well show more emphasis on health food outlets and self-medication.

☐ Problems of excessive vitamin intake

Vitamins are necessary for numerous metabolic reactions, but are needed only in small amounts. Taken in large quantities, they may cause chemical imbalances and one vitamin may interfere with the body's ability to use another (Luke 1985). In large quantities or with chronic usage, certain vitamins may be toxic.

The Committee on Medical Aspects of Food Policy (1991) notes the potential toxicity of vitamins A, thiamin, niacin, B_6 and C. Of even greater concern than this, are putative teratogenic effects − notably of vitamin A. Luke (1985) believes vitamin A to be one of the most dangerous non-prescription drugs available on the market.

Reports on the teratogenicity of vitamin A caused the concerns over self-medication with high dose vitamin preparations raised by Best *et al* (1989) as described above. Vitamin A occurs as carotene, which has not been associated with toxic effects, and retinol, which has (Teratology Society 1987). Evidence on the teratogenicity of vitamin A in humans remains equivocal due to a lack of epidemiological studies. However, there is much information indicating a need for extremely cautious use during pregnancy. This includes evidence from animal studies and case reports of fetal abnormalities following exposure to high doses of vitamin A (Rosa *et al* 1986; Teratology Society 1987). These abnormalities are similar to the widely recognised pattern of major malformations occurring after exposure to the drug isotretinoin (a synthetic analogue of vitamin A), used for treatment of acne. Various reports in the Lancet (Rosa 1983, Braun *et al* 1984; Lancet 1985) detail fetal abnormalities including microcephaly, hydrocephaly, microtia, microphthalmos, congenital heart disease and cleft palate. Lammer and colleagues (1985), in their study on retinoic acid embryopathy, report an 18 per cent risk of major malformations after exposure to isotretinoin during the first trimester. Craniofacial, cardiac, thymic and central nervous system structures were particularly affected.

Concern over vitamin A was further fuelled in 1990, when the then Chief Medical Officer, Sir Donald Acheson, issued a press release warning pregnant women, and those who were likely to become pregnant, not to take any supplements containing vitamin A, except on medical advice. He also cautioned against eating liver or liver products due to their high retinol content. It has been argued that this advice may be unnecessarily alarmist and based on very limited evidence of risk (Nelson 1990). Concern is also raised about inadequate dietary intake of vitamin A in the absence of liver, especially among lower socioeconomic groups (Nelson 1990; Saunders 1990). Whether or not the advice was alarmist, it serves to emphasise the fact that inappropriately high levels of vitamins may be harmful. Health care professionals and the general public alike, need to be aware of the potential dangers.

□   **The prevention of neural tube defects**

Over the years much has been written on the potentially protective action of vitamins against neural tube defects. Smithells *et al* (1981), having failed to obtain ethical approval for a double blind placebo trial, set up a multicentre intervention study. They gave a multivitamin preparation to women who already had a baby with a neural tube defect and who were planning a further pregnancy. The women started supplementation at least 28 days before conception, and continued until they had missed two periods. A non supplemented group comprised women who had previously given birth to babies with neural tube defects and who were pregnant again at the time of referral. Results indicated that vitamins could prevent some neural tube defects, but which specific vitamins were beneficial was unclear. Many questions were left unanswered due to the limitations of the design of this study and the results have since been contested.

Molloy *et al* (1985) compared serum folate and vitamin B_{12} concentrations for mothers with pregnancies affected by neural tube defects and randomly selected controls. They used serum samples that had been collected for routine rubella antibody screening, which were stored for 10 months after analysis at the laboratory in question. No significant differences were found between the two groups; 21.9 per cent of samples from the neural tube defect group and 22.8 per cent of control samples were deficient in either folate or vitamin B_{12}. The authors suggested that defective closure of the neural tube could take place in the presence of normal circulating values of the vitamins. They postulated that folate deficiency may be neither the main nor the sole cause of neural tube defects and that if it is involved it may be due to decreased availability to the fetus. They therefore indicated a need for further work on maternal transfer and fetal uptake of the vitamins.

Mulinare *et al* (1988) set out to discover whether or not there is a protective effect of periconceptual vitamin use among women who have not had a previous pregnancy affected by neural tube defects. Their survey used data from the Atlanta Birth Defects Case-control Study. The case group comprised all mothers who had given birth to live or stillborn babies with anencephaly or spina bifida. A control group of randomly selected mothers of healthy babies was matched to the group. The women were interviewed retrospectively about their use of periconceptual vitamins. A further control of mothers who had had babies with birth defects other than neural tube defects was selected to account for recall bias. Fourteen per cent of them had used vitamins during the entire six month period in question: 7 per cent of the case mothers and 15 per cent from the control groups. No use of vitamins was reported by 39 per cent (46 per cent of case mothers and 39 per cent of the controls). The results showed an apparently protective effect of periconceptual multivitamins which was statistically significant for white women but not for women of other races. The authors noted that whilst the risk of neural tube defect was different between those who took vitamins and those who did not, it was not possible to identify whether this was due to the vitamins or to other characteristics of the vitamin users.

The retrospective nature of this study, which relied on recall from as much as 16 years previously in some cases, has led to questions about the validity of the results. Mills and colleagues (1989) attempted to overcome these problems by interviewing women within five months of diagnosis of neural tube defect or delivery. Their study had a matched design similar to that of Mulinare *et al*, involving groups of women who had babies with neural tube defects and two control groups as described previously. It was still retrospective, however, and (like the study by Mulinare *et al*) involved women whose vitamin use was self-selected. Unlike Mulinare *et al*, Mills and colleagues found that women who had babies with neural tube defects were not less likely to have taken vitamin supplements and no significant association with folate use was identified.

These and other studies reaffirmed the need for a randomised trial. In 1983 the Medical Research Council set up a randomised double blind prevention trial involving thirty-three centres in seven countries. One thousand eight hundred and seventeen women who were at risk of having a baby with a neural tube defect because of a previous affected pregnancy were randomly allocated to one of four supplementation groups: folic acid, other vitamins, both or neither (MRC Vitamin Study Research Group 1991). By April 1991, sufficiently conclusive results had emerged to end the trial, before the target of 2000 pregnancies had been reached.

The prevalence of neural tube defects amongst the group receiving folic acid was one per cent; amongst those not receiving it, 3.5 per cent. There was no indication that vitamins other than folic acid had any preventative effect. No adverse effects of supplementation were identified, but follow up of the children involved is continuing. The authors concluded that 72 per cent of neural tube defects were prevented by supplementation with folic acid. Six women had babies with neural tube defects despite being supplemented with folic acid. The authors note that serum folic acid concentrations were not unusually low in these women. They do not believe that lack of compliance or failure of absorption are likely reasons, but offer no further explanation. The possibility of heterogeneous aetiology has been suggested elsewhere (Lancet 1991). The authors recommended that all women with a previous affected pregnancy should be offered folic acid supplements and that every effort should be made to ensure that women of childbearing age receive adequate dietary folic acid.

■ Conclusions

It is axiomatic that vitamins and minerals are essential dietary components and, as such, play an important role in pregnancy. It does not necessarily follow, however, that augmenting their levels with medication is always a good thing. A discussion of all the available research on supplementation is outside the scope of this chapter, but the examples used serve to highlight some of the issues with an important bearing on practice. These may be summarised as follows.

Routine prophylaxis with iron and vitamins is favoured by some authors, but general agreement is that it is unnecessary. Controversy remains over when it is appropriate to give supplements. The level at which alteration in serum nutrients in pregnant women ceases to be physiological and becomes indicative of deficiency has not been established. Until further research identifies acceptable parameters, pregnant women will continue to be treated as abnormal variants of the non-pregnant population.

The work on iron levels in pregnancy exemplifies the problem. There is a marked decline in iron stores beginning quite early in pregnancy, probably in response to erythropoiesis. Minimal stores are left when fetal requirements are greatest. This occurs irrespective of supplementation, but the work of Foulkes and Goldie (1982) suggests that women with serum ferritin levels above 50 microgram/l at booking are unlikely to become anaemic during pregnancy. Absorption of iron is low while stores are being depleted but increases later when fetal requirements are significant. Thus stores become the limiting factor for red cell mass expansion (Murphy *et al* 1986). Given the problems related to high haemoglobin levels outlined above, attempting to boost haemoglobin with supplements at this time is of dubious value. If the reduction in stores was in response to deficiency, one would expect absorption to be increased. The fact that most women refill their stores by six weeks postpartum without supplements suggests that their net haemoglobin is adequate; furthermore, several authors report a lack of subjective improvement in health to mothers from taking supplements (Hytten & Leitch 1971; BMJ 1978; Bentley 1985).

Whilst unnecessary *prescription* of iron is at issue, inappropriate *self-medication* with vitamins is more a cause for concern. Tablets formulated with pregnancy in mind are unlikely to cause harm, but some other preparations, available for instance at health food shops, are less safe. In particular, high doses of vitamin A are potentially teratogenic. Education is needed on these dangers. It is often assumed that 'health food means natural means good', but it must be remembered that vitamin and mineral supplements are drugs with corresponding benefits and hazards.

Considering this, the discrepancy found by Best *et al* (1989) between vitamin use as recorded in the notes and that indicated by interview is a cause for concern. Luke (1985) discusses the importance of careful assessment at booking of both diet and supplement use, so that proper advice can be given. If we are failing in this, women may be taking inappropriate supplements unaware of potential dangers.

The Medical Research Council work on vitamins and the prevention of neural tube defects indicates that folic acid has a significant role to play. It emphasises the need for good periconceptual nutrition. Several authors point to the fact that blanket prescription of supplements diverts attention away from the importance of diet. Hemminki and Starfield (1978) comment on the psychological stress caused by side effects of supplements and the depressing effect this has on appetite. Smail (1981) believes supplementation to be an easy answer to nutritional problems which would be better solved by education. Midwives are already well placed to provide much of the necessary education during their encounters with mothers but need to establish means of reaching more women preconceptually (see Shorney 1990).

Routine supplementation with iron and vitamins has been described as a 'ritual' costing millions of pounds (Hawkins 1981). The importance of supplements in promoting the health of certain at risk groups is not denied, but subjecting all women to them irrespective of need diverts attention away from the normality of childbirth, to the potential detriment of mother and baby.

■ Recommendations for clinical practice in the light of currently available evidence

1. Routine supplementation with iron and vitamins is unnecessary.

2. Considered assessment of iron status is important – screening serum ferritin levels at booking would enable those at risk of deficiency to be identified.

3. Women who have had a pregnancy affected by a neural tube defect should be offered folic acid supplements periconceptually.

4. Only supplements specifically intended for use in pregnancy should be taken. High dosage preparations should definitely be avoided.

5. Careful assessment should be made at booking of dietary habits and supplement use.

6. Every opportunity should be taken to promote good nutrition and healthy eating.

■ Practice check

- What advice is given in your area on the need for iron and vitamin supplements?

- What criteria are used to define the need for supplements?

- How effective are your questioning techniques at eliciting relevant and accurate information?

- Do you make the most of your health education opportunities on diet and nutrition?

■ References

Bennett C, McIlwaine G 1985 A study of antenatal vitamin and iron supplementation in Glasgow. Health Bulletin 43 (4): 182–6

Bentley D 1985 Iron metabolism and anaemia in pregnancy. In Letsky E (ed) Clinics in Haematology 14 (3): 613–28

Best A, Little J, Macpherson M 1989 Vitamin supplementation in pregnancy. Journal of the Royal Society of Health 109 (2): 60–63

Braun J T, Franciosi R A, Mastri A R, Drake R M, O'Niel B L 1984 Isotretinoin dysmorphic syndrome. Lancet i: 506–7

British Medical Journal 1978 Editorial: Do all pregnant women need iron? British Medical Journal 2: 1317

Chesley L C 1972 Plasma and red cell volumes during pregnancy. American Journal of Obstetrics and Gynecology 112: 440–50

Committee on Medical Aspects of Food Policy 1991 Dietary reference values for food energy and nutrients for the United Kingdom: a report of the Panel on Dietary Reference Values of the Committee on Medical Aspects of Food Policy. HMSO, London

Department of Health 1990 Women cautioned: watch your Vitamin A intake. DoH, London (18.10.1990)

Drug and Therapeutics Bulletin 1984 Rational use of vitamins. Drug and Therapeutics Bulletin 22 (9): 33–6

Fenton V, Cavill I, Fisher J 1977 Iron stores in pregnancy. British Journal of Haematology 37: 145–9

Foulkes J, Goldie D 1982 The use of ferritin to assess the need for iron supplements in pregnancy. Journal of Obstetrics and Gynaecology 3: 11–16

Hawkins D 1981 Routine iron in pregnancy – is it necessary? Modern Medicine August 1981: 12

Hemminki E, Starfield B 1978 Routine administration of iron and vitamins during pregnancy: review of controlled clinical trials. British Journal of Obstetrics and Gynaecology 85: 404–10

Hytten F 1985 Blood volume changes in normal pregnancy. In Letsky E (ed) Clinics in Haematology 14 (3): 601–12

Hytten F 1990 Nutritional requirements in pregnancy: what should the pregnant woman be eating? Midwifery 6 (2): 93–8

Hytten F, Leitch I 1971 The physiology of human pregnancy, 2nd edn. Blackwell Scientific Publications, Oxford

Kelly A, MacDonald D, McNay M 1977 Ferritin as an assessment of iron stores in normal pregnancy. British Journal of Obstetrics and Gynaecology 84: 434–8

Koller O 1982 The clinical significance of haemodilution during pregnancy. Obstetrical and Gynaecological Survey 37: 649–52

Koller O, Sandvei R, Sagen N 1980 High haemoglobin levels during pregnancy and fetal risk. International Journal of Obstetrics 18: 53–6

Lammer E, Chen D, Hoar R, Agnish N, Benke P, Braun J, Curry C, Fernhoff P, Grix A, Lott I, Richard J, Sun S 1985 Retinoic acid embryopathy. New England Journal of Medicine 313 (14): 837–41

Lancet 1985 Editorial: Vitamin A and teratogenesis. Lancet i: 319–20

Lancet 1991 Editorial: Folic acid and neural tube defects. Lancet 338: 153–4

Luke B 1985 Megavitamins and pregnancy: a dangerous combination. American Journal of Maternal-Child Nursing 10 (1): 18–23

Medical Research Council Vitamin Study Research Group 1991 Prevention of neural tube defects: results of the Medical Research Council vitamin study. Lancet 338: 131–7

Mills J, Rhoads G, Simpson J, Cunningham G, Conley M, Lassman M, Walden M, Depp O, Hoffman H 1989 The absence of a relation between the periconceptual use of vitamins and neural tube defects. New England Journal of Medicine 321 (7): 430–35

Molloy A, Kirke P, Hillary I, Weir D, Scott J 1985 Maternal serum folate and vitamin B_{12} concentrations in pregnancies associated with neural tube defects. Archives of Disease in Childhood 60: 660–65

Mulinare J, Cordero J F, Erickson J D, Berry R J 1988 Periconceptual use of multivitamins and the occurrence of neural tube defects. Journal of the American Medical Association 260 (21): 3141–5

Murphy J, O'Riordan J, Pearson J, Newcombe R, Coles E 1986 Relation of haemoglobin levels in 1st and 2nd trimesters to outcome of pregnancy. Lancet i: 992–4

Nelson M 1990 Vitamin A, liver consumption, and risk of birth defects. British Medical Journal 301: 1176

Rosa F W 1983 Teratology of isotretinoin. Lancet ii: 513

Rosa F W, Wilk A L, Kelsey F O 1986 Teratogen update: Vitamin A congeners. Teratology 33: 355–64

Saunders T 1990 Vitamin A and pregnancy. Lancet   336: 1375
Shorney J 1990 Preconception care – the embryo of health promotion. In
    Alexander J, Levy V, Roch S (eds) Antenatal care: a research-based approach
    (Midwifery Practice, Vol 1). Macmillan, Basingstoke
Smail S 1981 Dietary supplements in pregnancy (editorials). Journal of the Royal
    College of General Practitioners   31: 707–12
Smithells R, Sheppard S, Schorah C, Seller M, Nevin N 1981 Apparent
    prevention of neural tube defects by periconceptual vitamin supplementation.
    Archives of Disease in Childhood   56: 911–18
Svanberg B 1975 Absorption of iron in pregnancy. Acta Obstetrica et
    Gynaecologia Scandinavica   Supplement 48: 1–27
Swinhoe D J, MacLean A B, Gibson B E 1989 Iron and folate supplements
    during pregnancy. British Medical Journal   298: 118–19
Teratology Society Position Paper 1987 Recommendations for Vitamin A use
    during pregnancy. Teratology   35: 269–75
Truswell S 1990 Who should take vitamin supplements? British Medical
    Journal   301: 135–6

■ Suggested further reading

Campbell D M, Gillmer M D G 1982 Nutrition in pregnancy. Proceedings of the
    tenth study group of the Royal College of Obstetricians and Gynaecologists,
    Royal College of Obstetricians and Gynaecologists, London
Committee on Medical Aspects of Food Policy 1991 Dietary reference values for
    food energy and nutrients for the United Kingdom: a report of the Panel on
    Dietary Reference Values of the Committee on Medical Aspects of Food
    Policy. HMSO, London
Medical Research Council Vitamin Study Research Group 1991 Prevention of
    neural tube defects: results of the Medical Research Council vitamin study.
    Lancet   338: 131–7
Mahomed K, Hytten F 1989 Iron and folate supplementation in pregnancy. In
    Chalmers I, Enkin M, Keirse J (eds) Effective care in pregnancy and
    childbirth: Vol 1, 301–17. Oxford University Press, Oxford
Montgomery E 1990 Iron levels in pregnancy, physiology or pathology? Assessing
    the need for supplements. Midwifery   6: 205–14

Chapter 3

Exercise and pregnancy

Gillian Halksworth

To exercise or not to exercise is a dilemma women are often faced with when they become pregnant, yet the advice and information they request is not always available. Women have become increasingly active in sports and aerobic programmes, enjoying the physical and psychological benefits exercise brings. Therefore, exercise has become a part of everyday life for many and women are naturally reluctant to interrupt their usual routine or forsake the benefits gained from exercise whilst they are pregnant. Yet, they may also be hesitant to continue for fear of harming their baby.

In the past women have sought the advice of health professionals, often with the resultant suggestions of 'caution' and 'to avoid fatigue' whilst pregnant. Such words, however, do little to reassure or guide the woman appropriately. Indeed fatigue can be induced by normal housework, yet there is little research investigating possible harmful effects of this everyday activity.

Lack of knowledge in the area of exercise and pregnancy could lead to a lost opportunity to promote a healthy lifestyle. Similarly, the current practice of inappropriate advice often given by some health professionals regarding exercise needs to be addressed.

This chapter seeks to explore some of the literature available and considers how exercise may affect the course of pregnancy, the development of the fetus and the health of the mother. There is also some brief discussion about the value of exercise during the puerperium.

■ It is assumed that you are already aware of the following:

- The normal anatomy and physiology of the human body;
- The adaptive changes of the human body in pregnancy;

- Normal exercise physiology (Wiswell 1991);
- The format and content of general relaxation and exercise sessions held in parentcraft classes.

■ Exercise and conception

Although exercise is generally found to be beneficial in terms of a healthy lifestyle and physical fitness (DoH 1992), little scientific evidence demonstrates conclusively the positive effects of physical activity on health. Yet the general consensus is that exercise is beneficial, the majority of people feeling both psychological and physical benefits (Bruser 1968; Katz 1985; Mellion 1985; Wolfe *et al* 1989; Fletcher 1991; Wiswell 1991). Intense exercise, however, may cause problems with the female reproductive system. In school years, it has been noted that there is a delay in breast development and menarche in girls who participate zealously in sporting activities. This is thought to be due to a reduced secretion of gonadotrophin-releasing hormone and hence, a decreased hormonal secretion by the ovaries (Hutton 1986; Drinkwater & Davajan 1991). The reason for the reduced secretion of gonadotrophin-releasing hormone has not been clearly identified. One theory suggested is that exercise induced production of β-endorphins and metenkephalins, two natural opioids, suppress its secretion (Russell *et al* 1985; Hutton 1986).

Similarly, Hutton (1986) suggests that menstrual irregularities occurring later in life can be associated with exercise. This applies to problems in the luteal phase of the ovulatory cycle as well as to anovulation and amenorrhoea.

The mechanisms by which physical activity affects the menstrual cycle are not clear. Physical conditions such as low body weight, common in athletes, was one theory, however, studies now question this suggestion (Russell *et al* 1984; Drinkwater & Davajan 1991). Similarly, dietary changes such as a high protein diet taken during training was thought to be responsible for hormonal changes and hence secondary amenorrhoea (Hutton 1986). However, there is no conclusive evidence for this and researchers are still trying to investigate a possible endocrine cause (Russell *et al* 1984; Drinkwater & Davajan 1991).

Russell *et al* (1984) found that β-endorphins and catechol oestrogens were significantly increased with exercise and can be related to the decrease in luteinizing hormone seen in the oligomenorrhoeic group in this study. Hutton (1986) considers that psychological factors, such as the stress of competitive sport, may also affect the menstrual cycle. Drinkwater & Davajan (1991) suggest that, as there is no clearly defined cause for these menstrual dysfunctions, it may be a combination of personal characteristics, lifestyle and hormonal responses to strenuous exercise. In order to conceive,

Drinkwater and Davajan (1991) suggest that the individual concerned should make moderate changes in dietary habits and exercise regime to encourage resumption of normal menses.

Hence, athletes often experience problems such as amenorrhoea or anovulatory cycles which can lead to difficulties in conceiving or failure to recognise pregnancy, resulting in late booking for antenatal care (Hutton 1986; Drinkwater & Davajan 1991).

■ Effects of antenatal exercise on pregnancy and labour

Once a woman is pregnant the changes in her reproductive system are supported by secondary changes and adjustments in other systems of the body. The anatomical changes of pregnancy such as laxity of joints and ligaments, together with increased weight and a continuous shift in the centre of gravity, may mean that pregnant women are more susceptible to injuries during exercise (Artal *et al* 1989; Artal *et al* 1990). Additionally, exercise is a physiological stressor which stimulates the body to make adjustments to cope with the demands being made. There is an increase in endocrine and neuromotor activity; heat production demands a modification of the normal mechanisms of thermoregulation; fluid and electrolyte balance is altered and fuel sources are demanded (Wiswell 1991).

The body normally copes with this stress and after training will perform well at different levels of exercise.

□ Preparation for labour

Physical conditioning can reduce the catecholamine response and increase the capacity of the aerobic system, hence exercise may be beneficial in preparing pregnant women for the physical and psychological stress of labour (Rauramo *et al* 1982; Russell *et al* 1984; Artal Mittlemark 1991). In particular, Varrassi *et al* (1989) demonstrated that physical conditioning during pregnancy increases β-endorphin levels. They found an inverse correlation between β-endorphin levels and pain perception. There was a significant reduction in pain perception as well as reduced stress levels during labour among those women who had taken regular exercise while pregnant.

Wiswell (1991) suggests that an individual's capacity for exercise is limited by the combined ability of the respiratory and cardiovascular systems to meet the increased oxygen demand of the muscles. The physiological symbol for oxygen consumption, VO_2, is a measure of cardiovascular endurance – representing as it does the relationship between heart rate and exercise intensity giving the percentage of the predetermined maximum oxygen consumption. In the resting state VO_2 is equivalent to basal metabolic rate: VO_2 maximum is defined as an individual's maximal rate at which oxygen can be utilised by the body. In theory VO_2 maximum is measurable when a person is exercising at maximum heart rate. In pregnancy VO_2 maximum is often unattainable because the physical changes limit a woman's ability to achieve this state of exertion. An individual prediction of the maximum oxygen uptake can be made from the heart rate response to submaximal work loads (Pomerance et al 1974; Kulpa et al 1987; Wiswell 1991). It is this prediction of VO_2 maximum which is often used in estimating maximal aerobic capacity in pregnancy.

With training the ability to utilise oxygen more efficiently at more demanding workloads with less cost to the cardiovascular system would improve an individual's aerobic capacity and hence will prepare and improve an individual's ability to tolerate labour (Dressendorfer 1978; Wilson & Gisolfi 1980; Morton et al 1985a; Kulpa et al 1987; Artal Mittlemark et al 1991a).

As gestation advances the metabolic cost of a given task increases. Different types of exercise have different effects however: non-weightbearing activities such as swimming and bicycling, which have less effect than exercises involving weightbearing activities such as running, may therefore be more advisable for some.

□ **Aquanatal exercise**

Non-weightbearing exercise may be the most appropriate method of exercise in pregnancy (Bruser 1968; Sibley et al 1981; Artal et al 1989; Durak et al 1990). The ultimate non-weightbearing exercise is that performed when immersed in water. Hence, researchers suggest that swimming may be the perfect aerobic activity for pregnant women (Sibley et al 1981; Katz 1985; Katz et al 1991).

Water has been recognised for its therapeutic properties since ancient times and similarly today hydrotherapy is a useful means to facilitate muscle development. Water aerobic activities cause less strain on the joints and the individual can enjoy mobility because of the buoyant effect of the water (Reid Campion 1990). Additionally concern about thermoregulation during exercise is reduced as the ability to eliminate heat is greater in water and the potential teratogenic effects caused by a rise in core temperature avoided (Katz et al 1991).

McMurray et al (1988) studied the effect of pregnancy on metabolic responses during rest, immersion and aerobic exercise in water. Their results suggest that although there were changes in the metabolic responses (for example blood glucose levels declined slightly during exercise, plasma cortisol concentrations remained lower during immersion and exercise, and blood triglyceride levels were elevated with exercise) these did not have any detrimental effects and therefore concluded that immersion and moderate exercise in water do not result in any metabolic compromise.

An important aspect of their study, however, was the temperature of the water. Normal swimming pools are usually heated to 25°C to 28°C, however, 30°C was found to be the most beneficial temperature for exercise programmes. Immersion for long periods in cooler water may result in heat loss and thermodiscomfort: exposure to water of less than 28°C will result in shivering in an attempt to maintain core temperature. Temperatures above 36°C will cause vasodilation and can limit a person's capacity to exercise. Therefore, the optimum temperature suggested for exercise is in water of 28–30°C.

During the studies by McMurray *et al* (1988) and Katz *et al* (1988, 1991) which were performed at 60 per cent VO_2 maximum, both maternal and fetal wellbeing were monitored. No cardiovascular compromise was found in either mother or fetus. Uterine activity was similarly unaffected. Fetal breathing motion, fetal movement and fetal awake state had a rhythmic variation suggesting no adverse fetal effect.

McMurray *et al* (1988) also found that maternal heart rate responses during immersion in water were less marked than those during land exercise. They attributed this result to the greater filling of the heart in response to hydrostatic pressure. The hydrostatic pressure of water exerts a force which acts uniformly on the body to push extravascular fluid into the vascular space resulting in a rapid expansion of plasma volume. As the intravascular volume increases a diuresis is initiated. Renal vascular resistance decreases and hence there is an increase in filtration. The study showed that immersion of women in water for 20–40 minutes results in a 300–400 ml loss in fluid while blood volume is maintained. The researchers postulate that immersion therapy could be used to alleviate symptomatic oedema in some women (McMurray *et al* 1988; Katz *et al* 1991).

The above effects of hydrostatic pressure are particularly related to water aerobic sessions, however, whether a similar extravascular fluid redistribution occurs during swimming is not clear. Swimming in a supine position causes some redistribution of fluid volume but because the body is not totally immersed, the effects of hydrostatic pressure will be less. Yet, most swimmers tend to adopt a vertical position at various times during the exercise session and therefore will benefit from the hydrostatic effect at these periods (Katz *et al* 1991).

With swimming during pregnancy there may be a potential problem of straining the lower back in the position commonly adopted for breast stroke. Most swimmers, when performing recreational breast stroke, swim with their head out of the water which tends to make the lower back overarch and, with the added weight of the pregnant abdomen, the lumbar lordosis is accentuated. Therefore, it is advisable either to perform the breast stroke with a stream line body keeping the head in the water or to use other strokes such as side or back stroke (Dale & Roeber 1987).

Immersion exercise appears to have many advantages over other sporting activities for pregnancy. Sibley *et al* (1981) noted that the women enjoyed psychological benefits from water exercise in the form of improved appetite; better sleep patterns and increased feeling of wellbeing. Water exercise is particularly suited to the overweight person, as obesity is not so noticeable in the pool and exercises which would be stressful on land are easily performed in water. The social aspect of group aquanatal classes can be psychologically beneficial for pregnant woman (Katz 1985; Balaskas & Gordon 1990).

☐ Exercise as treatment for gestational diabetes

Although studies in this area are limited, there is a suggestion that cardio-vascular conditioning programmes, such as aerobic exercise, may prevent the need for insulin treatment in women with gestational diabetes. Using an upper body exercise programme while measuring stress by means of an arm ergometry machine, Jovanovic-Peterson and Peterson (1991) found that exercise facilitated glucose utilisation by increasing insulin binding with its receptor, thereby preventing the need for insulin therapy. Other studies have been performed with similar results (Artal *et al* 1989; Wolfe *et al* 1989).

☐ Psychological aspects

It is suggested by many that exercise is not only physically beneficial in terms of muscular development, physical fitness, and relieving some of the minor disorders of pregnancy, but it also enhances a sense of wellbeing and improved self-esteem (Sibley *et al* 1981; Mellion 1985; Wallace *et al* 1986; Hall & Kaufman 1987; Noble 1988; Williams *et al* 1988; Wolfe *et al* 1989; Artal & Artal Mittlemark 1991). Improving self-confidence at an emotionally vulnerable time in a woman's life can only be positive.

Wallace and colleagues (1986) used the Rosenberg self-esteem scale to compare the psychological wellbeing and the incidence of physical discomforts in women participating in aerobic exercise during pregnancy. The exercising group of women had statistically significant higher self-esteem and lower physical discomfort scores than the group of women who did not exercise. In particular there was a lower incidence in the exercise group of physical symptoms of backache, shortness of breath, fatigue, headache and hot flashes.

Hall and Kaufman (1987) also studied the effects of a physical conditioning programme on pregnancy outcome and the subjective pregnancy experience. Hence, in addition to the birth outcome, the exercising group were surveyed to evaluate self-image, any reductions in physical discomforts of pregnancy, relief of tension and speed of recovery. All those exercising reported improved self-image and a decrease in physical discomforts during the time of participation. Additionally, those who continued their conditioning programme until term felt that the exercise programme was beneficial in preparing them for labour and delivery. Furthermore, the multiparous women felt that recovery was more rapid than after previous pregnancies.

Mellion (1985) discusses the view that exercise is an effective therapy for people who are anxious or depressed. He suggests that 'exercise produces a sense of mastery and control, and the positive effects of being successful in an exercise programme spill over into other realms of life'.

■ Exercise and the fetus

Although carefully regulated exercise may be beneficial (as discussed above) the dangers of too much exercise or the wrong sort of exercise should not be overlooked. In particular, exercise which causes changes to the cardiovascular or thermoregulatory systems may put the fetus at risk.

□ Blood flow redistribution during exercise

During exercise blood volume shifts from the internal organs (splanchnic vessels) to the working muscles and skin: the shift increasing with the intensity of the exercise. Other cardiovascular responses include increases in cardiac output (heart rate, stroke volume and systolic blood pressure) (Anderson 1987; Hale 1987; Wallace & Engstrom 1987; Huch & Erkkola 1990). In theory, therefore, the cardiovascular responses to exercise could cause placental insufficiency and fetal hypoxia as the blood flow to the pregnant uterus and intervillous space may be reduced.

Whether uterine blood flow during exercise is maintained at sufficient levels to satisfy the needs of the fetus has not been conclusively demonstrated as yet. Some researchers (Lotgering *et al* 1984; Spatling *et al* 1992) postulate that, although a reduction in uterine blood flow suggests a reduction in the supply of oxygen and nutrients to the uterus, this may not happen in practice. A marked rise in maternal haematocrit is associated with exercise: plasma filtrate is forced across the capillary membrane in exercising muscles resulting in a decrease in plasma volume while the red blood cell mass remains constant. This is associated with an increase in haemoglobin concentrate and hence an increase in blood oxygen carrying capacity. Therefore, the suggested reduced blood flow to the uterus during exercise may not cause a significant loss in oxygen delivery. Additionally, the blood flow within the uterus may compensate by favouring the placental cotyledons at the expense of the myometrium ensuring sufficient and constant oxygen availability to the fetus.

Suggestions have also been made that exercise could trigger preterm labour in some (Artal *et al* 1981) and in others exercise could adversely influence the growth rate of the fetus (Veille *et al* 1985; Douglas *et al* 1987; Manshande *et al* 1987; Artal Mittlemark & Posner 1991).

Various studies have been undertaken to assess these potential problems. In any study, however, researchers have to take into account the fact that response to exercise is very individual and affected by factors such as the age, weight and physical condition of the individual. Similarly, the type and duration of the exercise and the environment in which the exercise is performed will affect the individual's response. Furthermore, there are technical difficulties in assessing the fetal heart rate while the mother is moving. Therefore, precise and accurate results are not easily obtained. Studies have been performed on pregnant animals (e.g. Orr *et al* 1972; Clapp 1980; Lotgering *et al* 1983) but it is questionable whether the results can be generalised to humans given the anatomical and physiological differences. Despite these limitations to some of the studies, interesting and relevant issues are raised.

Lotgering *et al* (1983) studied uterine blood flow at different levels (percentage of maximal oxygen consumption) and duration of exercise in sheep. They found that vigorous exertion reduced uterine blood flow and fetal arterial oxygen tension and may have produced significant fetal hypoxia but this was impossible to test accurately. However, these particular results were from pregnant ewes who were exercised to the point of maternal exhaustion! Therefore, Lotgering and colleagues concluded that uterine blood flow was inversely related to the intensity and duration of the exercise.

In another study (Orr *et al* 1972), the results suggested that uterine blood flow did not change during intense treadmill exercise in pregnant ewes. The same study also suggested that blood diversion from the uterus was less when they had undergone training.

Clapp (1989a) studied the effects of exercise performed by women during early pregnancy. The results suggested that continuation of previously performed exercise is not associated with an increased incidence of spontaneous abortion or of any other abnormal first trimester event. The study also demonstrated that in physically fit women, activity between 50–85 per cent VO_2 maximum ability preconceptually and during early pregnancy does not significantly alter early pregnancy outcome. Similarly, Hale and Artal Mittlemark (1991) state that there is no data to suggest that physical activity can induce a spontaneous abortion.

Pijpers *et al* (1984) studied the effects of short term moderate maternal exercise on the human maternal and fetal cardiovascular system using Doppler ultrasound techniques. The results suggested that immediately following moderate short term maternal exercise there are no cardiovascular signs of fetal stress. Similarly, Carpenter and colleagues (1988) found that fetal heart rate was not affected through submaximal maternal exercise which was up to 70 per cent of maximal aerobic capacity (maternal heart rate less than or equal to 148 beats per minute). However, maximal maternal exertion was followed by fetal bradycardia, suggesting inadequate fetal gas exchange. Collings and Curet (1985) also studied fetal heart rate through a programme of exercise during the course of the pregnancy. The results demonstrated that the fetal heart rate accelerated after maternal exercise but the rates were within the normal or moderate tachycardia range with no evidence of fetal bradycardia. Additionally, the neonatal findings were such as to suggest that fetal growth and development was not affected when the mother exercised up to approximately 70 per cent of her maximal capacity. As suggested above attempting maximal capacity may lead to fetal hypoxia.

Some studies suggest that there may be a redistribution of blood flow within the uterus to compensate for the apparent reduced blood flow during exercise (Oakes *et al* 1976; Collings *et al* 1983; Lotgering *et al* 1983; Jovanovic *et al* 1985; Sady *et al* 1990). Further work is still needed however.

□ **Catecholamines**

One cause of fetal hypoxia could be excessive catecholamine production associated with maternal stress, either physical as with exercise or psychological (Douglas *et al* 1987). Uterine vasculature is sensitive to catecholamines, hence the mechanism for blood flow redistribution is mediated by these catecholamines. Plasma catecholamine levels increase during exercise and the amount of the increment depends on the intensity and duration of the exertion (Zuspan *et al* 1962; Artal *et al* 1981; Rauramo *et al* 1982; Platt *et al* 1983). These studies have shown that pregnant women respond to exercise programmes with significant increases in both epinephrine and norepinephrine which can cause hypoxia in the fetus. Yet, neonatal findings of those experiencing intense exercise programmes do not substantiate these theories (Zuspan *et al* 1962; Jarrett & Spellacy 1983; Collings & Curet 1985). Indeed, Dibblee and Graham (1983) found that Apgar scores were higher in the exercise group in their study. It can also be argued, however, that physical conditioning can decrease the catecholamine response to a given exercise stress and hence avoid any potential problems such as fetal hypoxia (Orr *et al* 1972; Winder *et al* 1978; Russell *et al* 1984).

Additionally, norepinephrine is known to stimulate myometrial action and could, theoretically, induce preterm labour (Zuspan *et al* 1962; Adamson *et al* 1971; Artal *et al* 1981). Other studies (Veille *et al* 1985; Clapp 1989a; Wolfe *et al* 1989) have not supported this theory, however, and certainly a study of pregnant Olympic athletes whose exercise programmes were intense did not reveal a higher than average incidence of preterm labour (Zaharieva 1972). Similarly, a study of jogging during pregnancy revealed no correlation between exercise and preterm labour (Jarrett & Spellacy 1983).

□ Thermoregulation

Maternal hyperthermia can be injurious to the fetus (Edwards 1967; Miller *et al* 1978). During exercise the heat produced by working muscles can rapidly elevate the core temperature of an individual if heat transfer to the environment is not equal to production (Huch & Erkkola 1990; Drinkwater & Artal Mittlemark 1991). In pregnancy the fetus is an additional source of heat thus compounding the problem.

If maternal core temperature reaches 39°C or above then there can be serious consequences for the fetus. Teratogenic effects can include anencephaly and neural tube defects (Miller *et al* 1978), also uterine blood flow can be decreased. Such decrease in blood flow, however, may not necessarily result in a decreased umbilical blood flow (Oakes *et al* 1976). A study of hyperthermia during gestation in guinea pigs demonstrated that defects were more common and more severe in those heated in early gestation than those heated in mid gestation to late gestation (Edwards 1967).

In order to avoid hyperthermia, therefore, moderation of the training programme (by reducing the intensity of the exercise) is recommended. Additionally, ensuring adequate hydration whilst exercising, wearing the appropriate clothes and acclimatising to any changes in the environment are useful precautionary measures.

□ Effects on birthweight

Some studies have been performed to assess the effects of heavy physical work by women during pregnancy (Tafari *et al* 1980; Prentice *et al* 1981; Manshande *et al* 1987). Results suggested that excessive maternal exertion did affect the birthweight and the avoidance of the same could improve the outcome. However, caution has to be taken when interpreting these results as the studies were undertaken in developing countries where nutritional factors may also have influenced the results.

In contrast, Hall and Kaufman (1987) found that in an industrial society birthweights were higher for babies of women in a high exercise group compared to those in the control. Similarly, other studies (Zaharieva 1972; Dibblee & Graham 1983; Collings & Curet 1985; Kulpa *et al* 1987) found that fetal growth and development were not affected by exercise during pregnancy.

The general consensus, however, appears to be that it is advisable to reduce the intensity of any exercise programme in the last trimester (Morton *et al* 1985b; Anderson 1987; Huch & Erkkola 1990). In relation to work, Hatch and Stein (1991) suggest that heavy lifting, prolonged standing and strenuous work late in pregnancy should be avoided.

■ Postnatal exercise

Recovery from pregnancy and delivery varies from individual to individual and depends to a certain extent on the mode of delivery. However, by six weeks the majority of physical and physiological changes made for pregnancy have been reversed (Balaskas & Gordon 1990; Artal Mittlemark *et al* 1991b). Gentle exercise can be resumed as soon as feasible after a normal delivery if desired, gradually resuming a programme of regular exercise once the woman is feeling fit and able to make arrangements for an exercise session (Dale & Roeber 1987; Noble 1988; Fletcher 1991).

It should be remembered that the effects of relaxin can persist for up to 12 weeks after the birth. Therefore, it is suggested that weightlifting and extreme stretching should be avoided for the first three months postnatally (Artal Mittlemark *et al* 1991b). Swimming and water exercise can be resumed following cessation of lochia and healing of any tissue damage (Katz 1985). There appears to be little effect of exercise on lactation providing adequate hydration is maintained; however, it may be advisable to breastfeed prior to an exercise session as there is a suggestion that the quality of the milk may differ after exercise (Artal Mittlemark *et al* 1991b).

■ Legal aspects

Little has been written about the legal aspects of midwives involved in exercise programmes. Liability is usually based on negligence whereby the practitioner must have failed in his or her duty and caused the patient harm (Gallup 1991; see also the chapter by Robert Dingwall in this volume).

A midwife's duty is to give the appropriate, 'supervision, care and advice to women during pregnancy, labour and the postnatal period' (UKCC 1991). Therefore, although there are few specific guidelines regarding exercise, appropriate advice should be given to enable the woman to make an informed decision about participating in activities. Exercise itself involves some risk but the increased risk of exercising in pregnancy should be discussed and appropriate modifications made to an individual's programme as necessary. Advice should be given on a one-to-one basis, and should involve assessment of the woman's health and fitness to undertake the exercise of her choice, as well as giving due consideration to the fetus.

Any pregnant woman presenting with serious medical or obstetric problems should probably be advised to avoid any exercise programmes to prevent further complications.

Midwives actually teaching exercise programmes should be appropriately prepared to lead the class and be fully aware of the potential problems. Gallup (1991) suggests that liability may ensue for failing to warn about environmental conditions. Hence, it is important to advise clients about potential dangers which may seem obvious, encouraging them to take care when leaving the swimming pool following an aquanatal class, preparing them for the difference between the seeming weightlessness due to the buoyant support felt in water and the additional weight they will feel when emerging onto dry land, and drawing their attention to any slippery side walking areas in the swimming pool. Adequate lifesaver coverage should be ensured too of course. Other aspects (discussed earlier) including the importance of adequate hydration and avoidance of hyperthermia/ hypothermia, should always be stressed before each exercise class.

In the event of a problem arising, good documentation is obviously vital. Concern about litigation should not prevent midwives becoming involved in exercise sessions, however. With careful planning and sensible programmes which adhere to appropriate safety precautions, a lot of fun and enjoyment can be gained for both mothers and midwives alike.

■ Conclusions

The available research suggests that mild to moderate exercise is not harmful to the healthy normal pregnant woman and fetus (Wallace *et al* 1986; Huch & Erkkola 1990; Artal Mittlemark *et al* 1991a). Indeed, it has been seen that there are many potential benefits to be gained from it. There is a suggestion, however, that some specific sporting activities are ill advised in pregnancy and that modifications to others should be made. Sporting activities advised against throughout pregnancy are scuba diving and contact sports such as basketball or hockey. As pregnancy advances and the centre of gravity shifts the potential for injury is increased. Therefore, sporting activities requiring particularly good balance and co-ordination – such as ice skating, horse riding, gymnastics, waterskiing and downhill skiing – may well be better avoided later in pregnancy (Hale 1987; Wallace & Engstrom 1987; Artal Mittlemark *et al* 1991b).

Laxity of the joints in pregnancy may make sprains and other joint or ligament injuries more likely. Weight lifting and weightbearing sporting activities may need to be adapted. Weight lifting activities should be modified as pregnancy develops, using very light weights to prevent ligamental and joint injuries particularly to the lower back (Artal *et al* 1986). Advice such as using soft running surfaces and well cushioned shoes are recommended to those keen to maintain running programmes. Racquet sports may cause problems later in pregnancy due to the loss of speed in manoeuvring because of increased size; playing with a partner in doubles may be less demanding and more suitable later in pregnancy. Aerobic workout programmes, which are weightbearing sessions, should be modified for pregnant women and the same precautions as previously stated apply regarding joint injuries, overextension and hyperthermia (Wallace & Engstrom 1987; Grez 1988; Williford *et al* 1989; Artal Mittlemark *et al* 1991b). Alternatively, it may be more advisable to alter exercise activities to low impact sports such as walking, bicycling, yoga or swimming. However, bicycling carries risks of falling and may strain the lower back due to the weight of the fetus and position adopted when riding a bicycle late in pregnancy. The benefits of swimming and aquanatal classes have already been discussed.

Yoga has many advantages over other activities in having both a relaxation effect and promoting muscle tone and flexibility. Some postures may have to be modified for pregnancy particularly in the later months. Those postures which involve a supine position should be avoided altogether in view of aortacaval occlusion; similarly, overstretching should also be avoided (Milner 1988; Artal Mittlemark *et al* 1991b; Weller 1991).

Exercise has a number of effects on the course of pregnancy and the developing fetus. Similarly, being pregnant affects the ability to exercise. However, as Lotgering and colleagues (1985) suggest:

> Although the demands of pregnancy might compete with those of exercise, under most circumstances, the maternal organism can meet the combined demands of exercise and gestation through a remarkable reserve of physiological adjustments.

■ Recommendations for clinical practice in the light of currently available evidence

1. Exercise is a daily aspect of life for many and it is important for midwives to be able to advise and support women appropriately to enable them to participate in safe physical activity.

2. Minimum standards should be set to ensure that adequate safety precautions are met to promote the health of mother and fetus during exercise sessions run by midwives.

3. Adequate training courses should be provided for midwives leading exercise sessions.

4. Further research is needed into the benefits and hazards of exercise in pregnancy, the effects of exercise training on labour and on recovery during the puerperium.

5. Clinical audits of exercise programmes should be established to evaluate the quality, effectiveness and suitability of the sessions in meeting clients' needs.

6. It is important to involve student midwives in exercise programmes to ensure continued promotion of exercise initiatives.

■ Practice check

- Is an exercise history taken as part of the initial antenatal booking procedure?

- Are you giving the appropriate advice to women who wish to continue to exercise during pregnancy in respect of suitable exercise sessions and necessary safety precautions?

- Is the knowledge base in your area appropriate to organise suitable exercise sessions (such as aquanatal classes) to meet the needs of clients? If there is not an adequate knowledge base or suitable skills available could an action plan be developed to address these issues?

- Are there alternative forms of up to date parentcraft classes in your area, catering for those with differing needs, or for those who did not partake actively in exercise before becoming pregnant but require some guidance during pregnancy and encouragement to participate actively after the birth?

□ Acknowledgements

Thanks are due to many, particularly Richenda Milton-Thompson for her patience and constant reassurance; Val Levy for all her continued support; Jean Keats and the midwifery tutors at East Glamorgan Hospital for all their seemingly never ending support and encouragement.

■ References

Adamsons K, Mueller-Heubach E, Myers R E 1971 Production of fetal asphyxia in the rhesus monkey by administration of catecholamines to the mother. American Journal of Obstetrics and Gynecology 109 (2): 248–62

Anderson T D 1987 Exercise and sport in pregnancy. Maternal and Child Health Feb 15 (Update Section): 346–52

Artal M, Artal Mittlemark R 1991 Emotional aspects of exercise in pregnancy. In Artal Mittlemark R, Wiswell R A, Drinkwater B A (eds) Exercise in pregnancy. Williams & Wilkins, Baltimore

Artal R, Masaki D I, Khodigviann N, Romem Y, Rutherford S, Wiswell R 1989 Exercise prescription in pregnancy: weight bearing versus non-weight bearing. American Journal of Obstetrics and Gynecology 161: 1464–9

Artal R, Friedman M J, McNitt-Gray JL 1990 Orthopedic problems in pregnancy. The Physician & Sports Medicine 18 (9): 93–105

Artal R, Platt L D, Sperling M, Kammula R, Jilek J, Nakamura R 1981 Maternal exercise: cardiovascular and metabolic responses in normal pregnancy. American Journal of Obstetrics and Gynecology 140: 123–7

Artal R, Wiswell R, Romem Y, Dorey F 1986 Pulmonary responses to exercise in pregnancy. American Journal of Obstetrics and Gynecology 154: 378–83
Artal Mittlemark R 1991 Hormonal responses to exercise in pregnancy. In Artal Mittlemark R, Wiswell R A, Drinkwater B A (eds) Exercise in pregnancy. Williams & Wilkins, Baltimore
Artal Mittlemark R, Wiswell R A, Drinkwater B A (eds) 1991a Exercise in pregnancy. Williams & Wilkins, Baltimore
Artal Mittlemark R, Wiswell R A, Drinkwater B L, St John Repovich W 1991b Exercise guidelines for pregnancy. In Artal Mittlemark R, Wiswell R A, Drinkwater B (eds) Exercise in pregnancy. Williams & Wilkins, Baltimore
Artal Mittlemark R, Posner M D 1991 Fetal responses to maternal exercise. In Artal Mittlemark R, Wiswell R A, Drinkwater B A (eds) Exercise in pregnancy. Williams & Wilkins, Baltimore
Balaskas J, Gordon Y 1990 Water birth. Unwin Hyman, London
Bruser M 1968 Sporting activities during pregnancy. Obstetrics and Gynecology 32 (5): 721–5
Carpenter M W, Sady S P, Hoegsberg B, Sady M A, Haydon B, Cullinane E M, Coustan D R, Thompson P D 1988 Fetal heart rate response to maternal exertion. Journal of the American Medical Association 259 (20): 3006–9
Clapp J F III 1980 Acute exercise stress in the pregnant ewe. American Journal of Obstetrics and Gynecology 136: 489–94
Clapp J F III 1985 Fetal heart rate response to running in mid-pregnancy and late pregnancy. American Journal of Obstetrics and Gynecology 153: 251
Clapp J F III 1989a The effects of maternal exercise on early pregnancy outcome. American Journal of Obstetrics and Gynecology 161: 1453–7
Clapp J F III 1989b Oxygen consumption during treadmill exercise before, during and after pregnancy. American Journal of Obstetrics and Gynecology 161: 1458–64
Collings C A, Curet L B, Mullin J P 1983 Maternal and fetal responses to maternal aerobic exercise program. American Journal of Obstetrics and Gynecology 145: 702–7
Collings C, Curet L B 1985 Fetal heart rate response to maternal exercise. American Journal of Obstetrics and Gynecology 151: 498–501
Dale B, Roeber J 1987 Exercises for childbirth. Century Hutchinson, London
Department of Health 1992 The health of the nation. A strategy for health in England. HMSO, London
Dibblee L, Graham T E 1983 A longitudinal study of changes in aerobic fitness, body composition and energy intake in primigravid patients. American Journal of Obstetrics and Gynecology 147: 908–14
Douglas C, Hall M D, Kaufmann D 1987 Effects of aerobic and strength conditioning on pregnancy outcomes. American Journal of Obstetrics and Gynecology 157: 1199–203
Dressendorfer R H 1978 Physical training during pregnancy and lactation. Physician & Sports Medicine 6: 74–80
Drinkwater B L, Davajan V 1991 Amenorrheic atlhelete and conception. In Artal Mittlemark R, Wiswell R A, Drinkwater B A (eds) Exercise in pregnancy. Williams & Wilkins, Baltimore
Drinkwater B L, Artal Mittlemark R 1991 Heat stress and pregnancy. In Artal

Mittlemark R, Wiswell R A, Drinkwater B A (eds) Exercise in pregnancy. Williams & Wilkins, Baltimore

Durak E P, Jovanovic-Peterson L, Peterson C M 1990 Comparative evaluation of uterine response to exercise on five aerobic machines. American Journal of Obstetrics and Gynecology 162 (3): 754–6

Edwards M J 1967 Congenital defects in guinea pigs following induced hyperthermia during gestation. Archives of Pathology 84: 42–4

Fletcher G 1991 Get into shape after childbirth. Ebury Press for the National Childbirth Trust, London

Gallup E 1991 Legal aspects of exercise prescription and pregnancy. In Artal Mittlemark R, Wiswell R A, Drinkwater B A (eds) 1991 Exercise in pregnancy. Williams & Wilkins, Baltimore

Grez S A 1988 Bend and stretch. Maternal and Child Nursing 13: 357–9

Hale R W 1987 Exercise and pregnancy: how each affects the other. Postgraduate Medicine 82 (3): 61–3

Hale R W, Artal Mittlemark R 1991 Pregnancy in the elite and professional athlete. In Artal Mittlemark R, Wiswell R A, Drinkwater B A (eds) Exercise in pregnancy. Williams & Wilkins, Baltimore

Hall D C, Kaufmann D A 1987 Effects of aerobic and strength conditioning on pregnancy outcomes. American Journal of Obstetrics and Gynecology 157 (5): 1199–203

Hatch M, Stein Z A 1991 Work and exercise during pregnancy: epidemiological studies. In Artal Mittlemark R, Wiswell R A, Drinkwater B A (eds) Exercise in pregnancy. Williams & Wilkins, Baltimore

Huch R, Erkkola R 1990 Pregnancy and exercise – exercise and pregnancy. British Journal of Obstetrics and Gynaecology 97: 208–14

Hutton J D 1986 Effect of exercise on puberty, periods and pregnancy. New Zealand Medical Journal 99 (794): 6–8

Jarrett J C II, Spellacy WN 1983 Jogging during pregnancy: An improved outcome? Obstetrics and Gynecology 61: 705–9

Jovanovic-Peterson L, Peterson C M 1991 Fuel metabolism in pregnancy – clinical aspects. In Artal Mittlemark R, Wiswell R A, Drinkwater B A (eds) Exercise in Pregnancy. Williams & Wilkins, Baltimore

Jovanovic L, Kessler A, Peterson C M 1985 Human maternal and fetal response to graded exercise. Journal of Applied Physiology 58: 1719–22

Jones R L, Botti J J, Anderson W M 1985 Thermoregulation during aerobic exercise in pregnancy. Obstetrics and Gynecology 65 (3): 340–5

Katz J 1985 Swimming through your pregnancy. Thorsons, Wellingborough

Katz V L, McMurray R, Berry M J, Cefalo R C 1988 Fetal and uterine responses to immersion and exercise. Obstetrics and Gynecology 72: 225–30

Katz V L, McMurray R, Cefalo R C 1991 Aquatic exercise during pregnancy. In Artal Mittlemark R, Wiswell R A, Drinkwater B A (eds) Exercise in pregnancy. Williams & Wilkins, Baltimore

Knuttgen H G, Emerson J R 1974 Physiological response to pregnancy at rest and during exercise. Journal of Applied Physiology 36 (5): 549–53

Kulpa P J, White B M, Visscher R 1987 Aerobic exercise in pregnancy. American Journal of Obstetrics and Gynecology 156: 1395–403

Langhoff-Roos J, Lindmark G, Kylberg E, Gebre-Medhin M 1987 Energy intake and physical activity during pregnancy in relation to maternal fat accretion and infant birthweight. British Journal of Obstetrics and Gynaecology 94: 1178–85

Lotgering F K, Gilbert R D, Longo L D 1983 Exercises in pregnant sheep: blood gases; temperatures and fetal cardiovascular system. Journal of Applied Physiology 55: 842–50

Lotgering F K, Gilbert R D, Longo L D 1984 The interactions of exercise and pregnancy. American Journal of Obstetrics and Gynecology 149: 560–8

Lotgering F K, Gilbert R D, Longo L D 1985 Maternal and fetal responses to exercise in pregnancy. Physiological Review 65: 1–36

Maeder E C 1985 Effects of sports and exercise in pregnancy. Postgraduate Medicine 77 (2): 112–14

Manshande J P, Eccels R, Manshande-Desmet V, Vlietinck R 1987 Rest versus heavy work during the last weeks of pregnancy: influence on fetal growth. British Journal of Obstetrics and Gynaecology 94: 1059–67

Maron M B, Wagner J A, Horvath S M 1977 Thermoregulatory responses during competitive marathon running. Journal of Applied Physiology 42: 909–13

Mellion M B 1985 Exercise therapy for anxiety and depression: 1. Does the evidence justify its recommendations? 2. What are the specific considerations for clinical application? Postgraduate Medicine: 77 (3): 59–98

McMurray R G, Katz V L 1990 Thermoregulation in pregnancy: implications for exercise. Sports Medicine 10 (3): 146–58

McMurray R G, Katz V L, Berry M J, Cefalo R C 1988 The effect of pregnancy on metabolic responses during rest immersion and aerobic exercise in the water. American Journal of Obstetrics and Gynecology 158: 481–6

Miller P, Smith D W, Shepard T H 1978 Maternal hyperthermia as a possible cause of anencephaly. Lancet 1: 519–21

Milner I 1988 Yoga for pregnancy and childbirth. Yoga and Life 4 (5): 4–6

Morton M J, Paul M S, Campos G R, Hart M V, Metcalfe J 1985a Exercise dynamics in late gestation: effects of physical training. American Journal of Obstetrics and Gynecology 152: 91–7

Morton M J, Paul M S, Metcalfe J 1985b Exercise during pregnancy. Symposium on medical aspects of exercise. Medical Clinics of North America 69 (1): 97–108

Noble E 1988 Essential exercises for the childbearing year. Houghton Mifflin, Boston

Oakes G K, Walker A M, Ehrenkranz R A, Cefalo R C, Chez R A 1976 Uteroplacental blood flow during hyperthermia with and without respiratory alkalosis. Journal of Applied Physiology 41 (2): 197–201

Orr J, Ungerer T, Will J, Wernicke K, Curet L B 1972 Effect of exercise stress on carotid, uterine and iliac blood flow in pregnant and non pregnant ewes. American Journal of Obstetrics and Gynecology 114: 213–17

Pijpers L, Wlandimiroff J W, McGhie J 1984 Effect of short term maternal exercise on maternal and fetal cardiovascular dynamics. British Journal of Obstetrics and Gynaecology 91: 1081–6

Platt L D, Artal R, Semel J, Sipos L, Kammula R K 1983 Exercise in pregnancy. American Journal of Obstetrics and Gynecology 147 (5): 487–91

Pomerance J J, Gluck L, Lynch V 1974 Physical fitness in pregnancy: its effect on pregnancy outcome. American Journal of Obstetrics and Gynecology 119 (7): 867–76

Prentice A W, Whitehead R G, Roberts S B, Paul A A 1981 Longterm energy balance in childbearing Gambian women. American Journal of Clinical Nutrition 34: 2790

Rauramo I, Anderson B, Loatikaimen T 1982 Stress hormones and placental steroids in physical exercise during pregnancy. British Journal of Obstetrics and Gynaecology 89: 921–5

Reid Campion M 1990 Adult hydrotherapy: a practical approach. Heinemann, London

Russell J B, Mitchell D, Musey P I, Collins D C 1984 The relationship of exercise to anovulatory cycles in female athletes: hormonal and physical characteristics. Obstetrics and Gynecology 63: 452–6

Sady M A, Haydon B B, Sady S P, Carpente M W, Thompson P D, Coustan D R 1990 Cardiovascular response to maximal cycle exercise during pregnancy and at two and seven months postpartum. American Journal of Obstetrics and Gynecology 162: 1181–5

Sibley L, Ruhling R O, Cameron-Foster J, Christensen C, Bolen T 1981 Swimming and physical fitness during pregnancy. Journal of Nurse-Midwifery 26: 3–12

Spatling L, Fallenstein F, Huch A, Huch R, Rooth G 1992 The variability of cardiopulmonary adaptation to pregnancy at rest and during exercise. British Journal of Obstetrics and Gynaecology 99 (Supplement 8) 1–40

Tafari N, Naeye R L, Gobezie A 1980 Effects of maternal undernutrition and heavy physical work during pregnancy on birth weight. British Journal of Obstetrics and Gynaecology 87: 222–6

Thistlewaite J 1989 Exercise in pregnancy: what advice should we give? Maternal and Child Health November 369–70

United Kingdom Central Council for Nursing, Midwifery and Health Visiting 1991 Midwives' Code of Practice. UKCC, London

Ueland K, Novy M J, Peterson E N, Metcalfe J 1969 Maternal cardiovascular dynamics: the influence of gestation age on the maternal cardiovascular response to posture and exercise. American Journal of Obstetrics and Gynecology 104 (6): 856–64

Varrassi G, Buzzano C, Edwards T 1989 Effects of physical activity on maternal plasma β-endorphin levels and perception of labour pain. American Journal of Obstetrics and Gynecology 160: 707–12

Veille J, Herhimer A R, Burry K, Speroff L 1985 The effect of exercise on uterine activity in the last eight weeks of pregnancy. American Journal of Obstetrics and Gynecology 151: 727–30

Wallace A M, Boyer D B, Dan A, Holm K 1986 Aerobic exercise maternal self-esteem and physical discomforts during pregnancy. Journal of Nurse-Midwifery 31 (6): 255–61

Wallace A M, Engstrom J L 1987 Effects of aerobic exercise on the pregnant woman and fetus and pregnancy outcome. Journal of Nurse-Midwifery 32 (5): 277–90

Weller S 1991 Easy pregnancy with yoga. Thorsons, London

Whiteford I H, Polden M 1984 Postnatal exercises. Courtesy Publishing, London

Williford H N, Scharff-Olson M, Blessing D L 1989 The physiological effects of aerobic dance. Sports Medicine 8 (6): 335–45

Williams A, Reilly T, Campbell I, Simherst J M 1988 Investigations of changes in responses to exercises and mood during pregnancy. Ergonomics 31 (11): 1539–49

Wilson N C, Gisolfi C V 1980 Effects of exercising rats during pregnancy. Journal of Applied Physiology 48: 34–40

Winder W M, Hagberg J M, Hickson R C, Ehisani A A, McLane J A 1978 Time course of sympathoadrenal adaptation to endurance exercise training in man. Journal of Applied Physiology 40: 725–8

Wiswell R A 1991 Exercise physiology. In Artal Mittlemark R, Wiswell R A, Drinkwater B A (eds) Exercise in pregnancy. Williams & Wilkins, Baltimore

Wolfe L A, Hall P, Webb K A, Goodman L, Monga M, McGrath M J 1989 Prescription of aerobic exercise during pregnancy. Sports Medicine 8 (5): 273–301

Zaharieva E 1972 Olympic participation by women. Journal of the American Medical Association 221 (9): 992–5

Zuspan F P, Cibils L A, Pose I V 1962 Myometrial and cardiovascular responses to alterations in plasma epinephrine and norepinephrine. American Journal of Obstetrics and Gynecology 84 (7): 841–51

■ Suggested further reading and resources

Artal Mittlemark R, Wiswell R A, Drinkwater B A (eds) 1991 Exercise in pregnancy. Williams & Wilkins, Baltimore

Dale B, Roeber J 1987 Exercises for Childbirth. Century Hutchinson, London

Fletcher G 1991 Get into shape after childbirth. Ebury Press for the National Childbirth Trust, London

Hughes H 1988 The complete prenatal water workout book. Avery, New York

Weller S 1991 Easy pregnancy with yoga. Thorsons, London

□ Exercise leaflet

YMCA Looking after your body before and after pregnancy. Available from London Central YMCA, 112 Great Russell Street, London WC1B 3NQ. Tel 071–580 2989

□ Posters

Antenatal and postnatal exercise wallcharts. Available from Chartex Products International Ltd, Unit 1, 20 Grasmere, Liden, Swindon, Wilts SN3 6LE

☐ **Video**

YMCA 1991 The Y Plan: Before and after pregnancy. Lifetime Vision Ltd. Available from Lifetime Productions International Ltd, Freepost 5 (WD4616), London W1E 4QZ

☐ **Training courses**

London Central YMCA, Training and Development Dept, 112 Great Russell Street, London WC1 3NQ

Chapter 4

Fetal medicine

Joanne Whelton

This chapter examines the development of fetal medicine, discusses issues concerning the ethical implications that may arise, and considers the role of the midwife within this field. Technological advances within obstetrics have led to the development of specific prenatal diagnostic techniques. Such techniques can be divided into those involving measurement of the chemicals in maternal blood, and invasive tests to remove tissues of fetal original.

The report of the Royal College of Physicians (1989) suggests that where parents understand the risk, the great majority will use whatever means available to them to avoid the birth of a seriously ill or handicapped child. The report advises that the goal of genetic and prenatal diagnostic provision must be to help these couples make an informed choice regarding both their own, and their family's future.

The development of techniques for prenatal screening has provided the means through which active prenatal management can also be attempted. Treatment of rhesus-isoimmunisation and some renal tract anomalies offer potentially successful outcomes in situations that may otherwise have resulted in a very poor prognosis.

The provisions of such care obviously require a highly skilled team of experts and a limited number of specialist fetal medicine departments have developed over recent years offering prenatal diagnosis and management.

■ It is assumed that you are already aware of the following:

- The principles of ultrasound and the midwife's role (Proud 1990);

- Basic embryology and fetal development;

- Basic genetics and patterns of inherited disease;

55

- Local policy within your own area regarding the availability of prenatal screening tests and counselling;

- Psychological aspects of pregnancy, grief and bereavement (Adams & Prince 1990; Prince & Adams 1990).

■ The development of prenatal diagnosis

As long ago as 1864, Aubinas attempted to view the fetus through transillumination of the mother's anterior abdominal wall with candle light and specially prepared black paper. But it was almost a century later before the first endoscopic visualisations were reported by Westin and Mori who, in the 1950s, tried to observe the fetus through the cervix, but with minimal success (Rodeck & Nicolaides 1983a).

☐ Ultrasonography

In 1955, Professor Iain Donald used metal flaw-detecting equipment to diagnose the differing ultrasonic characteristics of excised fibroids. His work, combined with that of two other pioneers in the field, Willcocks and Campbell, led to the use of high resolution real time scanners that we know today (Campbell 1983). Whittle (1991) suggests that as many as 90 per cent of women in the United Kingdom currently undergo an ultrasound examination at some time in their pregnancy. The vast majority of these examinations are in the early weeks to establish dates and viability, or in later pregnancy to determine fetal size or placental site. He also suggests that, in the view of some, the stage has now been reached when a routine anomaly scan may be considered almost mandatory to confirm or establish dates and viability.

The objectives of ultrasound screening are to assist in the reduction of perinatal mortality and morbidity. The majority of anomalies occur in apparently low risk groups and Whittle (1991) advises that universal screening is the only method by which these can be identified. Luck (1992) suggests that when routine scanning is performed at 19 weeks gestation with the availability of termination, perinatal morbidity and mortality can be reduced.

Whilst attempting to identify the effectiveness of routine ultrasonography in detecting fetal structural abnormalities in a low risk population, Chitty and colleagues (1991) concluded that, although it is successful, it can present several dilemmas in counselling. These dilemmas occur from findings such as mild dilatation of the fetal renal pelvis, or transient choroid plexus cysts, which may or may not be indicators of underlying chromosomal anomaly. The dilemma results from the question then raised as to whether to pursue genetic investigations. In consequence the parents may face considerable anxiety and the fetus be put at risk by an invasive procedure in order to investigate observed structural deviations from the 'normal range', which, if unassociated with an underlying chromosomal defect, may not present complications following birth.

A second objective of screening is to identify those fetuses with the need for *in utero* treatment. These cases usually take the form of shunting procedures and will be considered later in the chapter.

The final objective is to identify conditions in the fetus that are amenable to neonatal surgery. Prior knowledge that the baby is abnormal but has an operable condition may confer some advantage, but there is no real evidence to confirm this. Whittle (1991) reports that a small personal survey of babies with anterior abdominal wall defects has failed to show any benefit from prenatal diagnosis. He suggests that the hypothesis that diagnosis would allow the selection of those cases best delivered by caesarean section has not been borne out. However the pre-delivery identification of such structural anomalies may be helpful in ensuring that appropriate paediatric facilities are available at time of delivery.

The optimum gestation for undertaking an anomaly scan is considered to be 18–20 weeks. Whittle quotes Rizzo, who in a personal communication, reported that his studies indicated that 40 per cent of abnormalities could be detected at 20 weeks compared with 15 per cent at 16 weeks. The type of anomaly has a significant influence as to when it is likely to be identified. The pathogenesis of some conditions is not clear, for example some cystic hygromas visualised during ultrasound examination resolve spontaneously prior to birth (Abramowicz *et al* 1989).

The extent of the ultrasonographer's experience has a part to play in the successful identification of some defects. Allan and colleagues (1991) reported an increased detection rate of hypoplastic left heart as consequence of the experience gained by those undertaking scans of the four chambers of the fetal heart.

The question as to the safety of ultrasound when used as a screening test during pregnancy has been raised on several occasions (Proud 1990). A recent study examining the school performance of 8–9 year olds suggested that the risk of having poor reading and writing skills was no greater for children whose mothers had received ultrasound scans during pregnancy than for those whose mothers had not (Salvesen *et al* 1992).

■ Invasive procedures

□ Amniocentesis

The breakthrough in the field of human genetics in the late 1950s provided the opportunity for screening human tissues for abnormalities of their chromosomal composition. Since the 1930s amniocentesis has been performed to introduce dye into the uterus to facilitate x-ray. It was not until 1967, however, that it was used for acquiring samples of amniotic fluid for genetic screening. Other indications for amniocentesis are for amniotic fluid alphafetoprotein and for assessment of rhesus disease (Rodeck & Nicolaides 1983b).

Since fetal karyotyping has been used to detect fetal chromosomal abnormalities in older mothers, there has been a dramatic expansion in the use of prenatal chromosome studies. Although older mothers were the major group known to be at high risk for fetal chromosomal disorder, they were having only 20–30 per cent of the chromosomally abnormal children. However, because primary aetiological factors involved in the conception of chromosomally abnormal fetuses (other than advanced maternal age, a previously affected child or a parental chromosomal anomaly) have not been identified we have to rely upon the development of screening methods in the recognition of abnormality. Serum biochemical parameters – especially the 'triple test' (the combined use of maternal history, her serum alphafetoprotein (AFP), unconjugated oestriol and human chorionic gonadotrophin levels in predicting the level of risk of Down's syndrome and neural tube defects) and the identification of structural markers on ultrasound scan are becoming increasingly important (Gosden 1991). The use of the 'triple test' has doubled the detection rate of Down's syndrome without increasing the proportion of women having amniocentesis (Wald *et al* 1992).

☐ **Fetoscopy**

As recently as the early 1970s ultrasound imaging was still of poor quality, so in an attempt to exclude suspected neural tube defects Scrimgeour (1973) used, with partial success, a 2.2 mm fibre optic endoscope introduced into the uterus at laparotomy for direct visualisation of the fetal spine. This indication for fetoscopic examination of the fetus quickly became replaced as Serum AFP testing was introduced and ultrasound imaging improved.

In 1984, Nicolaides and colleagues wrote that the only means of prenatally excluding conditions such as mandibulofacial dysostosis was using this invasive procedure of fetoscopy. (The word derived from the Latin *fetus* and the Greek *episkopion* meaning 'to inspect'.) But today's improvements in the manufacture of scanning equipment enables such diagnoses to be made and confirmed using this non-invasive screening method alone.

Prior to Scrimgeour's attempts at fetoscopy, transabdominal endoscopy had been used in 1967 to perform intraperitoneal transfusions of hydropic fetuses who were victims of rhesus isoimmunisation. The procedure was complex and difficult to carry out, but identified the potential for enabling fetal blood sampling, intrauterine photography and intravascular fetal blood transfusion.

☐ Placentacentesis

Reports of fetal blood being obtained through 'blind' needling (i.e. placenta-centesis) began to appear (Kan 1974). Blood samples enabled a more rapid diagnosis than amniotic fluid. Such samples, however, were frequently contaminated with maternal blood and amniotic fluid. As they were not pure fetal blood, only a limited selection of diagnoses could be obtained by this method. It was primarily the haemoglobinopathies (i.e. sickle cell disease and thalassaemia) that were diagnosed in this way. When fetal plasma was required (e.g. for clotting studies) diagnosis was not possible. Fetal loss through blind needling occurred in as many as 7–10 per cent of the cases (Rodeck & Nicolaides 1983).

☐ Fetoscopic blood sampling

In 1978 Rodeck and Campbell documented the percutaneous use of a 1.7mm rigid fibreoptic endoscope to obtain a pure sample of fetal blood by puncturing an umbilical cord vessel. This instrument was very small in diameter and therefore the procedure, involving penetration through the maternal abdominal wall and uterus under local anaesthesia, carried less risk.

Rodeck and Nicolaides (1983a) recommended the optimal time for anatomical examination of the fetus using fetoscopy to be 15–18 weeks, as the amniotic fluid is clear and the relatively small size of the fetus made orientation easier. These authors recommend fetal blood sampling be delayed until 18–20 weeks, reporting that if it is undertaken any earlier the umbilical blood vessels appeared to bleed more easily and also the fetal blood loss was proportionately greater. While describing this development Whelton (1985a, 1985b) cited the common indications for fetal blood, skin and liver sampling at the time, and considered the specific role of the midwife in supporting and caring for parents undergoing such investigations.

☐ Ultrasound guided needling

With the continued improvement of ultrasound equipment the use of the fetoscope has ceased. Today fetal examination can be undertaken by ultrasound alone, while blood sampling is performed by ultrasound guided needling. Due to the smaller size (20–21 gauge) of the needle the risk of causing an associated amniotic fluid leak or spontaneous abortion is less than with fetoscopy. The spontaneous abortion rate may vary slightly according to the experience of those carrying out the procedure, but is commonly cited as 0.5–1 per cent (similar to that of amniocentesis) compared with that of 1–2 per cent associated with fetoscopy. The main

Table 4.1 Current common indications for fetal blood sampling (adapted from the work of Nicolaides 1991)

Indication	Examples
Inherited blood disorders	Sickle cell disease
	Haemophilia
Possible fetal infection	Toxoplasmosis
	Rubella
Karyotyping	Failed or ambiguous amniocentesis culture
	Fetal malformation
Small for gestation fetuses	For acid-base status
Rhesus isoimmunisation	For assessment/management
Thrombocytopenia	For diagnosis
	For assessment/management

indicators for fetal blood sampling in the 1990s are summarised in Table 4.1.

☐ · **Chorionic villus sampling (CVS)**

The recent applications of DNA techniques to the analysis of placental biopsy material has made it possible to diagnose many of congenitally inherited conditions during the first trimester. Fetal blood sampling is still necessary, however, for those patients for whom first trimester sampling is not possible; for example those who lack key relatives necessary for familial genetic analysis, and for those who require rapid fetal karyotyping in the second or third trimester.

The development of transcervical CVS offered a number of advantages:

... the sample obtained is fetal tissue and is therefore genetically and chromosomally identical to the fetus;
... it is accessible during the first trimester by a natural passage, i.e. the cervical canal;
... it can be obtained without perforation of the membranes around the fetus;
... the parents may benefit because there is less delay, termination of pregnancy if indicated is simple, and the physical and psychological traumas of second trimester termination are avoided.

(from Rodeck 1985)

Transcervical CVS is the traditional method of chorionic villus sampling and the first attempts at this method were made in 1974 (Hahnemann). The method of acquiring a sample of chorion frondosum is either by aspiration through a cannula or by biopsy using forceps. In a pregnancy greater than 12 weeks gestation, a transabdominal approach is used as tissue is more accessible via this route.

☐ Evaluation of CVS/amniocentesis

In an attempt to compare CVS with amniocentesis undertaken at 15–16 weeks, the Medical Research Council (1991) carried out a multi-centred European trial. Women seeking karyotyping of the fetus were randomly offered either CVS or amniocentesis and the outcomes were then examined. In those women undergoing the earlier CVS screening, there was a higher fetal loss rate, an increased number of terminations for chromosomal anomalies and more neonatal deaths. The neonatal death rate was associated with a higher number of very immature liveborn infants in this group. More diagnoses of abnormal chromosomes were made in the CVS group, mostly being trisomy 18 and mosaicism. Despite these findings, however, the report recognises that women will continue to request CVS because of the early screening it offers despite the additional risks compared with amniocentesis.

Evaluation of the risk of pregnancy loss following villus sampling before 12 weeks, as compared with loss following amniocentesis at 15–18 weeks, is made difficult due to the higher incidence of spontaneously occurring abortion within the first trimester. It may not be possible to determine those abortions that may have occurred prior to 12 weeks whether CVS was undertaken or not (Leading Article, *Lancet* 1991).

The need for a procedure which offers the least invasive technique, and therefore least risk to the pregnancy, whilst reliably offering the most accurate result has led to many dilemmas. An alternative has been sought by those attempting early amniocentesis. Rooney *et al* (1989) evaluated the use of amniocentesis for karyotyping carried out between 8–14 weeks of pregnancy (earlier than traditionally performed). Their research was an attempt to evaluate the reliability of culture of amniotic fluid at that stage of pregnancy. They concluded that there was 100 per cent success rate with those samples taken between 12–14 weeks. However, the impact of early amniocentesis upon the fetus especially in relation to lung development was not evaluated as all the pregnancies were planned terminations. Their findings were also supported by the MRC study which concluded by proposing that the use of early amniocentesis may indeed provide an additional option for prenatal screening, providing that comprehensive research is undertaken into the associated risks of this earlier test.

There have been reports from the United Kingdom of congenital limb abnormalities in infants following CVS (Firth *et al* 1991). North American reports, however, were compared with data derived from the British Columbian Congenital Malformations Registry to conclude that there was no increase in frequency of limb reduction defects in early CVS cases compared

with the population frequency (Leading Article, *Lancet* 1991). Such occur-
ances may be associated with the procedure being carried out by single
needle transabdominal aspiration before nine weeks gestation.

The understanding of DNA and its links with genetic disorders is no
longer the mystery it used to be. It is anticipated that the entire human
genome will be mapped and all the important genes sequenced by the year
2000 (Kingston 1989). Early prenatal diagnosis is now available for a
number of conditions including cystic fibrosis, Duchenne muscular dystro-
phy and Huntington's chorea.

■ Fetal medicine and intrauterine management

While most medical or correctable surgical abnormalities that can be diagnosed *in utero* are best managed by appropriate therapy after delivery at
term, for certain conditions continuation of the pregnancy may have a
progressively harmful effect upon the fetus. If the fetus is too immature
for delivery, intrauterine therapy becomes necessary in order to stop the
destructive consequences of the underlying defect while allowing fetal
growth and development to continue.

Ho (1988) describes a number of intrauterine procedures reported in
American journals as being undertaken in attempt to treat pathological
conditions such as hydrocephaly, hydronephrosis and tachyarrhythmias.
Many of these are still being evaluated and questions have been raised as to
the success of these interventions, especially with regard to the British
experience of attempted management of hydronephrosis. In 1983, the Fetal
Medicine and Surgery Society was established and produced a series of
guidelines for consideration prior to therapy (Manning *et al* 1984). The
Society highlighted the need for careful selection of those fetuses who were
identified as being appropriate for treatment, and that such decisions should
involve all those who may be concerned with the infants' care both before

Table 4.2   Indications for fetal therapy

Indication	Management
Rhesus disease	Intraperitoneal transfusion Intravascular transfusion
Obstructive uropathy	Vesico-amniotic shunt
Fetal cysts	Needle puncture and drainage
Unexplained fetal hydrops	Abdominal paracentesis Thoracocentesis
Fetal deficiency states (e.g. platelets)	Intravascular transfusion

and after delivery. Initial investigation into possible underlying chromosomal defect or extent of pre-existing damage of tissues is essential and parents must be made aware that such management is still experimental.

☐ Rhesus isoimmunisation

The incidence of rhesus haemolytic disease has diminished greatly since the widespread use of immunoprophylaxis. The disease is unlikely to be eradicated completely, however, as some women become sensitised during their first pregnancy and others due to mismatched transfusions or insufficient anti-D being given to cover a large feto-maternal haemorrhage. The aim of the management is to anticipate the impact of the maternal antibodies upon the fetus and to offer intrauterine fetal transfusions to prevent the fetus becoming anaemic and at risk of death as a consequence. Assessment of the fetus at risk is made from the history, quantitation of the mother's antibodies, the bilirubin concentration of amniotic fluid and, ultimately, fetal blood sampling.

Fetal blood sampling and intrauterine transfusions can be carried out as early as 18 weeks gestation. Seriously affected fetuses may receive a series of transfusions at two to four week intervals, depending on the rate of fall of the haemoglobin concentration which may be indicated by oedema indicative of hydrops fetalis developing. Group O rhesus negative red cells carrying blood group antigens that do not react with the maternal antibody are used, with a high packed cell content to achieve the minimum total volume load and the maximal correction of anaemia. Transfusions are usually given intravascularly via the umbilical vein for immediate correction and may be combined with intraperitoneal administration following which the blood is slowly absorbed through the lymphatics (Letsky 1990).

The use of serial intravascular transfusions has increased the survival rate of severely affected pregnancies. Success rates of between 78–90 per cent have been reported in severely affected fetuses (Rodeck & Fisk 1991).

☐ Obstructive uropathy

Of all organ systems the genito-urinary tract has the highest incidence of congenital abnormalities (Rodeck & Nicolaides 1983b). In fetuses where an obstruction is present at, or distal to, the urethro-vesical junction (e.g. posterior urethral valves) conditions, such as dilatation of the bladder, hydroureters, hydronephrosis and oligohydramnious, may result that are unassociated with other anomalies. The two main factors determining perinatal outcome are pulmonary hypoplasia and renal dysplasia (Harrison *et al* 1982).

The standard method of vesico amniotic shunting is by ultrasound guided insertion of an indwelling plastic double pigtail catheter that drains the urine from the distended fetal bladder into the amniotic cavity. This decompression of the urinary tract prevents further renal destruction and restores the amniotic fluid volume thus preventing the sequelae of oligo-hydramnios (failure of lung maturity, talipes and congenital hip disloca-tion). The results of 73 cases of shunting procedures for low obstructive uropathy reported to the International Registry were not encouraging, with only a 41 per cent perinatal survival rate (Manning *et al* 1986). Rodeck and Fisk (1991) consider that much of the scepticism about this procedure can be related to poor case selection. They suggest that if careful criteria for selection are used (excluding those cases with abnormal karyotype, severe oligohydramnios or inadequate renal function) management is likely to be successful.

☐ **Fetal hydrothorax**

Perinatal mortality in cases of fetal hydrothorax exceeds 50 per cent. Rodeck and Fisk (1991) suggest that there may be a congenital condition similar to that of chylothorax (pleural effusion) which is the commonest cause of hydrothorax in neonates. Their management of eight fetuses, which involved a drain being inserted, produced a successful outcome in six cases.

☐ **Intrauterine growth retardation**

Nicolini and colleagues (1990) reviewed the value of assessing fetal acid base status in relation to growth retardation. Their observations combined with those of biophysical profiles and Doppler studies suggest that these fetuses adopt a 'hibernation' state as a means of coping with the hypoxia that they experience. They concluded that the risks of fetal blood sampling outweigh the value of the information acquired. Campbell and Soothill (1990) dispute this, however, arguing that blood gas analysis may have a very important part to play in the reduction of prenatal brain damage.

■ **Psychological considerations**

The availability of prenatal screening has changed the experience of preg-nancy (Katz Rothman 1988). Prior to such tests for fetal abnormality, the fetus was assumed to be healthy, unless there was evidence to the contrary (Marteau 1991). The presence of prenatal testing and monitoring shifts the balance towards having to prove the health or normality of a fetus. Prenatal testing provides a much wanted choice for some prospective parents, particularly those at known risk of having a child with severe abnormality. Some parents will only embark on pregnancies knowing that testing and termination of affected fetuses is available, yet for other parents this is a choice they would prefer not to confront. Green (1990) suggests that the availability of prenatal diagnosis has opened the doors that cannot be closed.

Whether or not women undergo prenatal screening depends on three main factors (Marteau 1991):

- Whether the test is available;

- The knowledge and attitudes of the health professionals consulted;

- The knowledge and attitudes of the women themselves.

There may be a danger that too many available tests result in confusion. Lilford (1989) suggests that excessive choice may be bewildering for parents.

The experience of some mothers who are awaiting prenatal screening is described by Katz Rothman (1988). She identified women who feel unable to respond positively to the fact that they are pregnant until their test results are known. She describes the period of waiting for these results as 'the tentative pregnancy', in that the waiting, combined with the knowledge of the risk of abnormalities, leads many mothers who undergo amniocentesis to claim not to experience fetal movements until the normal result is confirmed at around 22–23 weeks. This impact may vary according to maternal age and the reasons for screening. In a study aimed at assessing anxiety levels, Tabor and Jonsson (1987) concluded that in younger women at low genetic risk amniocentesis was neither anxiety-relieving, nor anxiety-creating. They appeared to experience a decrease in anxiety once the procedure was over however, whilst for older women this did not occur until the results were available.

The factors that influence a woman's decision with regard to maternal serum alpha-fetoprotein (MS-AFP) and amniocentesis differ. For the blood test Marteau (1991) lists knowledge of the test, attitude to termination and perceived reliability of the test as significant considerations. Whereas for the woman considering amniocentesis, the perceived risk of having an affected child, attitude to termination and fear of miscarriage as result of the invasive procedure, are her suggested three priorities.

Women are generally ill informed about the tests that they are being offered. Using a self-administered questionnaire Marteau (1991) discovered that 39 per cent of women recently having had blood taken for MS-AFP were unaware that they had even had the test.

The increasing knowledge offered through screening tests can be a double edged weapon (Downe 1990) in that prenatal diagnosis may be a heavy burden to bear for both the parents and the midwives who may be involved with their care. Downe feels that 'we must begin to recognise that the power to choose life or death is a terrible one that carries profound psychological trauma'.

■ Ethical considerations

There are many ethical issues that arise from within prenatal diagnosis and fetal medicine. A major concern facing all midwives is that most women will be offered an anomaly scan around 18–20 weeks. It is as much the responsibility of the midwife to explain about the scan being a diagnostic process, as it is to explain the implications of blood tests (Whelton 1990). The midwife may be required to answer a woman's questions and to recognise her option to decline any of the tests she is offered. But what if the mother refuses fetal therapy for her baby? We are then faced with the bizarre situation of fetal versus maternal rights (Ho 1988). Whilst considering the rights of the fetus, Carter (1990) identifies that the acknowledgment of a new group's rights may conflict with and threaten the rights of an existing group.

Cases of disabled children sueing their parents for failing to seek prenatal diagnosis have already occurred in the United States. Questions have to be asked about the morality of bringing a severely disabled child into the world and about what level of fetal abnormality or what likelihood of disability justifies termination of pregnancy (Harris 1991). Two further crucial questions arise: 'What should we screen for?' and 'What should we do about what we find?' If Beethoven's mother had been pregnant today screening tests would have identified her fetus as being at risk of congenital syphilis. In view of this she may have opted to have a termination in order to save her child from the unpleasant symptoms (including the deafness that was to afflict him) which might develop.

Harris (1991) clearly explains that to believe it right to abort a fetus is not to be necessarily committed to the view that the world would be better off without that individual, nor that the individual would eventually wish that she/he had never been born, nor that the individual will be unhappy, nor that the individual would suffer. Nor, in aborting an individual in the circumstances faced by Beethoven's mother are we in any sense aborting a potential Beethoven. He reminds us that in all cases what we are aborting is actually a fetus and the rights and wrongs of that are determined by a consideration of the moral status of the fetus.

The author has seen handicapped siblings of fetuses undergoing prenatal diagnosis who are aware that, if their parents had known about their condition at a similar stage, they too may have been aborted. Black and Furlong (1984) propose that any counselling undertaken prior to prenatal screening should raise the issue of the impact upon siblings should the pregnancy be terminated. Their findings suggest that children are commonly already involved in the pregnancy and that its loss, for whatever reason, results in a crisis for the entire family.

Controversy exists over the right of the parents to be told the sex of their unborn baby. Policies as to whether to tell or not vary between hospitals, as well as between ultrasound and cytogenetic departments on occasions. Do health care professionals have the right to decide as to whether the information, if available, should be withheld from a mother who may be very keen to know? There are several obvious difficulties in accurately diagnosing the sex by ultrasound scan alone, however all karyotype cultures will reveal the presence of an x or y chromosome. Sadler (1991) offers a comprehensive discussion of reasons for and against divulging the sex from scan. The main problem identified is that ultrasonographers are afraid of litigation should they make an error. Not all women want to know the sex of their baby and this appears to be the reason that cytogenetic laboratories tend not to identify the fetal sex in the karyotype result as it will be filed in the mother's notes and may then be inadvertently disclosed.

The impact of the mother's knowledge of the infant's sex before delivery upon her attachment with her baby was examined by Grace (1984). She found that it had no ultimate influence upon 'bonding behaviour', and concluded that the option of being told the sex if determined during screening should be available for those who want it.

The impact of facing termination for fetal abnormality is described by Statham (1987). Sharing her personal experience she highlights the need for supportive counselling during such a life event. The provision of support after termination of pregnancy for abnormality has not proceeded at the same rate as the advances in prenatal diagnosis (Lloyd & Lawrence 1985). These authors suggest that the following are still needed:

• Better liaison between all those health care professionals involved with the mother;

• Organisation of support and counselling similar to that offered following perinatal loss;

• Genetic counselling to be offered where appropriate;

• Training of hospital and community based staff with regard to meeting the families' needs.

When a woman decides to terminate an abnormal fetus where is the best place for her care to be given? Should the termination take place on a gynaecological ward, or a labour ward (Whelton 1990)? These are questions we need to consider.

■ Counselling

Following the experience of termination of pregnancy for fetal anomaly, any subsequent pregnancy inevitably brings with it a great deal of stress. If adequate support was given after the previous loss the parents will be aware of the help that will be available in the future.

Couples should be encouraged to grieve the loss of that particular baby (Adams & Prince 1990) and seek genetic counselling for insight as to future risks. Genetic counselling aims to enable the parents to comprehend the medical aspects of diagnosis, possible cause and management. It also explains the hereditary implications and recurrence risks with the options for dealing with the same. An appropriate course of action can be agreed, planning care for any affected family member and/or for the risk of future pregnancies (Donnai & Kerzin-Storrar 1991). Clarke (1991) feared that it might be difficult for counselling to be non-directive in a clinical situation. Hence it may be necessary to refer parents for specialist counselling support or to put them in touch with other agencies such as the relevant religious group or self help organisation.

A question frequently asked is 'how soon can we try again?' This is not necessarily an attempt to replace the lost baby, but may be a need to prove that as parents they are not failures, and that they still have the ability to produce the child they were hoping for. It may be helpful to suggest to parents that they will need time to grieve (Adams & Prince 1990). It is important to remember too that if a woman falls pregnant shortly after the loss her expected date of delivery may coincide with the anniversary of the bereavement − which may be very stressful.

Prenatal diagnosis is here to stay. As health professionals caring for parents who are concerned to prevent the birth of a handicapped child, our duty is not to be judgemental. Rather, we must offer all parents the support and care they need whilst undergoing prenatal diagnosis and making difficult decisions.

■ Recommendations for clinical practice in the light of currently available evidence

1. There is a need for midwives involved with the care of mothers undergoing any type of prenatal screening to be aware of the specific tests involved, and the risks and implications of such tests.

2. Parents need to be more active participants in the decision about what prenatal screening, if any, to undergo.

3. Parents need to be given more information about the implications of ultrasound scans and tests such as MS-AFP. They should also be made aware of the risks involved in invasive prenatal screening.

4. Written information should be available explaining the following (Marteau 1991):

    - Purpose of testing;
    - Conditions screened for;
    - Likelihood that an abnormality will be detected;
    - The test procedure, including any risks;
    - Meaning of the results, both positive and negative;
    - Possible actions following a positive result.

5. Midwives caring for women and their partners who are facing the dilemmas of prenatal diagnosis must take responsibility for developing the self-awareness, integrity and tolerance that will enable them to give the best possible support and care to parents.

6. Midwives involved with parents experiencing termination of a fetus with an abnormality, themselves require a support network within the work environment.

■ Practice check

- Are you aware of the prenatal diagnostic provision within your health authority?

- Does your unit provide information sheets about the available tests? If not, do you consider that such sheets should be available? Can you suggest a draft format?

- Do you feel able to discuss with women the implications of prenatal diagnosis?

- As a midwife have you had the opportunity to sit in on a genetic counselling session? If not can you arrange to do so?

- Does your unit have standards of care for women undergoing termination of pregnancy for fetal abnormality?

- Does your unit have a staff support network? If not should you consider trying to set one up?

□ Acknowledgement

Thanks to Professor Charles Rodeck with whom I've worked for so many years.

■ References

Abramowicz J S, Warsof S L, Doyle D L, Sith D, Levy D L 1989 Congenital cystic hygroma of the neck diagnosed pre-natally; outcome with normal and abnormal karyotype. Prenatal Diagnosis 9: 21–7

Adams M, Prince J 1990 Care of the grieving parent with special reference to stillbirth. In Alexander J, Levy V, Roch S (eds) Antenatal care: a research-based approach (Midwifery Practice, Vol 1). Macmillan, Basingstoke

Allan L D, Cook A, Sullivan I, Sharland G K 1991 Hypoplastic left heart syndrome: effects of fetal echocardiography on birth prevalence. Lancet 337: 959–61

Black R B, Furlong R 1984 Prenatal diagnosis: the experience in families who have children. American Journal of Medical Genetics 19: 729–39

Campbell, S 1983 Foreword. In Clinics in Obstetrics and Gynaecology, Volume 10, No 3 (Ultrasound in Obstetrics and Gynaecology). WB Saunders, Eastbourne

Campbell S, Soothill PW 1990 Role of fetal blood gas analysis in intrauterine growth retardation (Letter). Lancet 336: 1316–17

Carter B 1990 Fetal rights – a technologically created dilemma. Professional Nurse 5 (11): 590–3

Chitty L, Hunt G, Moore J, Lobb M 1991 Effectiveness of routine ultrasonography in detecting fetal structural abnormalities in a low risk population. British Medical Journal 303: 1165–9

Clarke A 1991 Is non-directive genetic counselling possible? Lancet 338: 998–1001

Donnai D, Kerzin-Storrar R 1991 Counselling after prenatal diagnosis. In Drife J O, Donnai D (eds) Ante-natal diagnosis of fetal abnormalities. Springer–Verlag, London

Downe S 1990 The price of progress. Nursing Times 86 (8): 26

Firth H V, Boyd P A, Chamberlain P, MacKenzie I Z, Lindenbaum R H, Hudson S M 1991 Severe limb abnormality after chorion villus sampling at 56–66 days gestation. Lancet 337: 762–3

Gosden C 1991 Fetal karyotyping using chorionic villus samples. In Drife J O, Donnai D (eds) Antenatal diagnosis of fetal abnormalities. Springer–Verlag, London

Grace J T 1984 Does a mother's knowledge of fetal gender affect attachment? Maternity and Childrens Nurse 9: 42–5

Gregg J 1987 Codes, conscience and conflicts: ethical dilemmas in midwifery practice. Midwives Chronicle 100 (1199): 392–5

Green J M 1990 Calming or harming? A critical review of psychological effects of fetal diagnosis on pregnant women. Occasional papers, Second series No. 2. Galton Institute, London

Hahnemann N 1974 Early prenatal diagnosis: a study of biopsy techniques and cell culturing from extra embryonic membranes. Clinical Genetics 6: 294–306

Harris J 1991 Ethical aspects of prenatal diagnosis. In Drife J O, Donnai D (eds) Ante-natal diagnosis of fetal abnormalities. Springer–Verlag, London

Harrison M R, Golbus M S, Filly R A 1982 Management of the fetus with congenital hydronephrosis. Journal of Paediatric Surgery 17: 728–42

Ho E 1988 The unborn patient. Nursing Times   84 (5): 38–40

Kan Y W, Valenti C, Carnazza V, Guidotti R, Reider R F 1974 Fetal blood sampling *in utero*. Lancet   1: 79–80

Katz Rothman B 1988 The tentative pregnancy: prenatal diagnosis and the future of motherhood.   Pandora, London

Kingston H M 1989 DNA analysis in genetic disorders. British Medical Journal 229: 170–4

Lancet 1991 Leading article: Chorion villus sampling – valuable addition or dangerous alternative? Lancet   337: 1513–15

Letsky E A 1990 ABC of transfusion: Fetal and neonatal transfusion. British Medical Journal   300: 862–6

Lilford R J 1989 'In my day we just had babies'. Journal of Reproductive and Infant Psychology   7: 187–91

Lilford R J 1991 Invasive diagnostic procedures in the first trimester. In Drife J O, Donnai D (eds) Ante-natal diagnosis of fetal abnormalities. Springer–Verlag, London

Lloyd J, Lawrence K M 1985 Sequelae and support after termination of pregnancy for fetal malformation. British Medical Journal   290: 907–9

Luck C 1992 Value of routine scanning at 19 weeks: a four year study of 8849 deliveries. British Medical Journal   304: 1474–8

Manning F A, Lilo N, Walzack M D and Members of the International Fetal Medicine and Surgery Society 1984 Report of the Fetal Medicine and Surgery Society meeting, Washington DC

Manning F A, Harrison M R, Rodeck C H, and members of the International Fetal Medicine and Surgery Society 1986 Catheter shunts for fetal hydronephrosis and hydrocephalus. New England Journal of Medicine   315: 336–40

Marteau T M 1991 Psychological implications of prenatal diagnosis. In Drife J O, Donnai D (eds) Ante-natal diagnosis of fetal abnormalities. Springer–Verlag, London

Medical Research Council working group on the evaluation of chorion villus sampling (MRC) 1991 Medical Research Council European trial of chorion villus sampling. Lancet   337: 1491–99

Nicolaides K 1991 Cordocentesis. In Drife J O, Donnai D (eds) Ante-natal diagnosis of fetal abnormalities. Springer–Verlag, London

Nicolini U, Nicolaidis P, Fisk N, Vaughan J, Fusi L, Gleeson R, Rodeck C H 1990 Limited role of fetal blood sampling in prediction of outcome in intrauterine growth retardation. Lancet   336: 768–72

Nicolaides K, Johansson D, Donnai D, Rodeck C 1984 Prenatal diagnosis of mandibulofacial dysostisis. Prenatal Diagnosis   4: 201–5

Prince J, Adams M 1990 The psychology of pregnancy. In Alexander J, Levy V, Roch S (eds) Antenatal care: a research-based approach (Midwifery Practice, Vol 1). Macmillan, Basingstoke

Proud J 1990 Ultrasound – the midwife's role. In Alexander J, Levy V, Roch S (eds) Antenatal care: a research-based approach (Midwifery Practice, Vol 1). Macmillan, Basingstoke

Rodeck C 1985 Fetoscopy and chorion biopsy. Current therapy in Neonatal-Perinatal Medicine   1985–1986: 84–9

Rodeck C H, Campbell S J 1978 Sampling pure fetal blood by fetoscopy in second trimester of pregnancy. British Medical Journal   2: 728–30

Rodeck C H, Fisk N M 1991 Intrauterine therapy. In Drife J O, Donnai D (eds) Ante-natal diagnosis of fetal abnormalities. Springer–Verlag, London

Rodeck C H, Nicolaides K H 1983a Fetoscopy and fetal tissue sampling. British Medical Bulletin 39 (4): 332–7

Rodeck C H, Nicolaides K H 1983b Ultrasound guided invasive procedures in obstetrics. Clinics in Obstetrics and Gynaecology 10 (3): 515–39

Rooney D E, MacLachlin N, Smith J, Rebello M T, Loeffler F E, Beard R W, Rodeck C, Coleman D V 1989 Early amniocentesis: a cytogenetic evaluation. British Medical Journal 229: 25

Royal College of Physicians 1989 Prenatal diagnosis and screening, community and service implications: a report. RCP, London

Sadler C 1991 The right to keep mum. Nursing Times 87 (30): 16–17

Salvesen K A, Bakketeig L S, Eik-Nes S H, Undheim J O, Okland O 1992 Routine ultrasonography *in utero* and school performance at age 8–9 years. Lancet 339: 85–9

Scrimgeour J B 1973 In Emery AEH (ed) Antenatal diagnosis of genetic disease. Churchill Livingstone, Edinburgh

Statham H 1987 Cold comfort. The Guardian, March 24, page 26

Tabor A, Jonsson M H 1987 Psychological impact of amniocentesis on low risk women. Prenatal Diagnosis 7: 443–9

Wald N J, Kennard A, Densem W, Cuckle H, Chard T, Butler L 1992 Antenatal maternal serum screening for Down's syndrome: results of a demonstration project. British Medical Journal 305: 391–4

Westin B 1954 Hysteroscopy in early pregnancy. Lancet 2: 872

Whelton J M 1990 Sharing the dilemmas: midwives' role in prenatal diagnosis and fetal medicine. Professional Nurse 5 (10): 514–18

Whelton J 1985a Development of fetoscopy. Nursing Mirror 160 (23): 29–30

Whelton J 1985b Sensitive counsel. Nursing Mirror 160 (24): 43

Whittle M J 1991 Routine fetal anomaly screening. In Drife J O, Donnai D (eds) Ante-natal diagnosis of fetal abnormalities. Springer–Verlag, London

■ Suggested further reading

De Crespinney L 1991 Which tests for my baby? Oxford University Press, Melbourne and Oxford

Gregg J 1987 Codes, conscience and conflicts: ethical dilemmas in midwifery practice. Midwives Chronicle 100 (1202) 392–5

Kuhse H, Singer P 1985 Should the baby live? The problem of handicapped infants. Oxford University Press, Oxford

Lewis M, Faed M J W, Howie P W 1991 Screening for Down's syndrome based on individual risk. British Medical Journal 303: 551–3

Sutton A 1990 Prenatal diagnosis: confronting the ethical issues. Lincare Centre for the study of ethics of health care, London

■ Useful address

SAFTA (Support after termination for fetal abnormality)
29–30 Soho Square
London W1V 6JB
071 439 6124

Chapter 5

The elderly primigravida

Louise Silverton

The term 'elderly primigravida' was first used in 1958 by the International Council of Obstetricians and Gynecologists to refer to women aged over 35 years who were embarking upon their first pregnancy (Tuck *et al* 1988). Such a rigid cut off point has been criticised by Kane (1967) who demonstrated that risk increases (and outcomes worsen) from a maternal age of 25 years onwards. A review of the literature, however, indicates that a wider range of definition is used. Some authors are interested in primiparous women aged over 30 (Vessey *et al* 1986; Barkan & Bracken 1987), whilst others have only followed up those women aged over 40 (Berryman & Windridge 1991a, 1991b). For this reason, this chapter has not adopted a rigid definition but states the range of ages examined in each particular circumstance.

Most older first time mothers are categorised as being at high risk of complications and are given care in a consultant obstetric unit. This chapter seeks to make a case for such women to be considered individually with the choice of carer and place of care being selected as appropriate and in accordance with the woman's wishes. It will examine the level of risk (if any) experienced by these older first time mothers and place this within the context of midwifery care and the role of the midwife. Finally the woman's adaptation to pregnancy and her experiences of childrearing are considered before a review of guidelines for good practice.

To categorise all older first time mothers – a very diverse group of women – as being at high risk of complications due to age alone is, according to Gaskin (1986: p. 16), '... to be practising a very crude and unscientific brand of obstetrics' especially where this is not supported by research (Mansfield 1986; Berryman & Windridge 1991a). This 'high risk' label may well be resented by the woman (Cario *et al* 1985) especially where she pays attention to her health and lifestyle. Indeed, Holz *et al* (1989) point out that, in the United States, educated older women embarking on their first pregnancy are more likely to seek alternatives to the hospital based, medically supervised care than is the norm in that country. Midwives as practitioners and champions of the normal seek to encourage and empower women during the processes of childbearing, but this can be hard to achieve with those who are labelled as being at high risk of complications regardless of their individual circumstances.

■ It is assumed that you are already aware of the following:

- The physiology of pregnancy;

- The more common deviations from normal in labour and the interventions needed to counter them.

■ Position of women

The changes in fertility patterns which have led to more women becoming pregnant for the first time at an older age may be due to the wider educational and career opportunities available to women today, together with differing personal expectations, more reliable contraception and a delay in marriage (Bureau of Census 1989). Women today have greater control than their mothers or grandmothers over whether and when to have children (Adams *et al* 1982).

In England and Wales the age specific fertility rate for women aged 35–39 years has increased from 18.2 births per 1000 women in 1977 to 31.7 in the year to June 1991 and that for women aged over 40 years from 4.4 to 5.3 (OPCS 1992). Although this does not show how many of these women are first time mothers, total first births in England and Wales to women aged 35–39 have increased from 3900 in 1976 to 9100 in 1990 and for those aged over 40 years from 700 to 1300 in 1990 (OPCS 1992), whilst births to older women of high parity have reduced. A similar trend has been noted in the United States with a doubling of first births to women aged 35–39 and a 50 per cent increase for those women aged over 40 years between 1970 and 1986 (National Center for Health Statistics 1989).

Midwives are likely to encounter the older first time mother in their practice, particularly where they give care to women of high socioeconomic status. Tuck and colleagues (1988) report an over representation of women from higher socioeconomic groups amongst primigravidae aged over 35 years who had been voluntarily childless until this time. When a profile of the older primipara is examined, she is more likely than younger women to be of higher socioeconomic status and married or in a stable relationship (Cario *et al* 1985). Robinson and colleagues (1987) showed that older primipara were less likely to hold traditional attitudes regarding women's roles in society than were younger women.

Given the increased expectation of life after 40 years of age, the woman and her partner can expect to live to see their offspring reach maturity and independence (Stein 1985) in a way that could not have been contemplated in the past. The delaying of a first birth is most common amongst more educated women (those who have completed schooling at 18 years and/or have had higher education) who tend to present early for care and either have or adopt a healthy lifestyle (Ventura 1982). It has been suggested by some authors that the adoption of a healthy lifestyle may well reduce (in some cases to a minimum) any effects of ageing (Davidson & Fukushima 1986; Lehmann & Chism 1987).

Stein (1985) suggests that it was the questioning climate of the late 1960s with its rejection of established values (such as early marriage and childbearing) that began the increase in voluntary childlessness and older first time childbearing. Daniels and Weingarten (1982) suggest that childbearing may be delayed because of the fear of the psychological and financial stresses and strains associated with pregnancy and childrearing. Such a decision may also be related to employment and home ownership.

The older first time mother adapts well to pregnancy and is usually a conscientious attender for antenatal care and parent education sessions (Stein 1985). However some women may worry about the 'high risk' label which has been applied to them and are concerned about the way in which medical advice favours childbearing at an earlier age (Mansfield & Cohn 1986). It is important for the midwife to raise and discuss such issues with the woman in order to prevent inappropriate anxiety.

■ What are the risks?

Evidence regarding the adverse effects of increasing maternal age on pregnancy outcome in primiparae is confusing and sometimes contradictory (Berkowitz *et al* 1990). A review by Mansfield (1986), of 104 studies conducted between 1912 and 1983, found serious flaws in the methodology of 61 per cent of the studies. Several studies included important variables other than age, and 29 per cent drew conclusions which did not derive from the data presented or which were backed up with insufficient statistics. Mansfield suggests that the adverse outcomes reported were more likely to be due to pre-existing disease, subfertility, high parity and unplanned pregnancy than to the biological effects of ageing. Other authors have also placed stress on the importance of pre-existing medical disorders which are exacerbated by increasing age (Adams *et al* 1982; Naeye 1983).

Tuck and colleagues (1988) state the importance of differentiating those women aged over 35 who have been voluntarily childless from those who have been experiencing infertility (see Table 5.1). Because of the potential difference in outcome they undertook to view these two groups of women

Table 5.1 Pregnancy outcome for older primigravidae with or without a history of subfertility or abortion when compared with primigravidae in a younger age group

		Low birth-weight	Preterm birth	Growth retardation	Perinatal mortality
Poland *et al* 1977 (women over 30)	History of abortion	+	+		
	No such history	ND	ND		
Barkan & Bracken 1987 (women over 30)	History of abortion or subfertility	+	+		
	No such history	ND	ND		
Tuck *et al* 1988 (women over 35)	History of subfertility	+	+	ND	
	No such history	+	+	ND	
Berkowitz *et al* 1990 (women over 35)		+	ND	ND	ND
Jonas *et al* 1991 (women over 35)		+	+		ND

Key + = increased risk; ND = no difference in outcome
(Where no information is given on a particular aspect, the relevant column is left blank)

separately in their retrospective study of pregnancy. Past obstetric history has an influence on outcome with an increase in preterm births and low birthweight being reported amongst older women with a history of sub-fertility (Barkan & Bracken 1987) and spontaneous abortion (Poland *et al* 1977). However, Barkan and Bracken (1987) have noted no increase in the occurrence of preterm birth or low birthweight amongst women aged over 30 with no history of subfertility or spontaneous abortion when compared to similar women aged less than 30. In contrast, whilst Jonas *et al* (1991) reported that primipara aged over 35 years had a greater incidence of both preterm birth and low birthweight, this was not reflected in a significantly raised perinatal mortality rate.

Tuck *et al* (1988) showed that primigravid women aged over 35 years (but with no history of subfertility) had a preterm delivery rate of 6.1 per cent when compared with 1.5 per cent for a matched group of 20–25 year olds. They had a low birthweight rate of 8.2 per cent compared with 3.6 per cent but there was no difference in the numbers of babies who were small for gestational age. In contrast, Berkowitz *et al* (1990) found that while women aged over 35 years were more likely than those aged 20–29 to give birth to a low birthweight infant, when socioeconomic factors were controlled for they had no increased risk of preterm birth, intrauterine growth retardation, low Apgar score or perinatal death. However these older women did have a greater risk of antenatal and labour complications, operative delivery and of the admission of their baby for neonatal intensive care. Mansfield (1986) in her review of studies highlighted an increase in perinatal mortality due to iatrogenic prematurity following elective operative births in some older mothers. This increase was, she felt, due more to anxiety on the part of the obstetricians than to other, genuine, indicators and might, therefore, have been avoided.

When looking at the occurrence of low birthweight, Lee *et al* (1988) demonstrated that the lowest incidence at term was in births to mothers aged 24–34 with the highest rates for births to 17 year olds and an increase after the age of 35 years which was more marked for women of higher parity. The authors suggest that the reduced potential for fetal growth is possibly related to biological ageing of either maternal tissues or biological systems or to the cumulative effect of disease. Kirz and colleagues (1985), however, found few statistically significant differences in outcome in their study of over 1000 primiparous women aged over 35 years compared with a control group aged 20–25 years. They attribute their 'success' to the high standard of care given in a tertiary care centre although, as with many such claims, there is little supporting evidence for this conclusion.

Maternal mortality increases with maternal age independently of parity. The maternal mortality rate in the United Kingdom for first time mothers aged 35–39 years between 1976–1987 was 282.8 per million maternities and 638.7 for those aged over 40. This compares with 65.3 per million for primipara aged 20–24 and an overall rate for all mothers of 86.7 per million (DoH 1991).

■ Complications of pregnancy and labour

□ Fertility

Edwards and Steptoe (1983) showed that following *in vitro* fertilisation both implantation failure and spontaneous abortion increase with maternal age. In a study (van Noord-Zaadstra *et al* 1991) of the outcomes of assisted reproduction in relation to maternal age, it was reported that the probability of giving birth to a healthy baby reduced by 3.5 per cent for every year of maternal age after the age of 30. The same study also looked at the effectiveness of artificial insemination by donor (AID) in relation to the age of the woman, the chances of success reduced after 31 years of age. After 12 treatment cycles a pregnancy had occurred in 74 per cent of women aged between 20–31 years and in 54 per cent of those over this age. After 24 treated cycles the difference was less at 85 per cent for the younger women and 75 per cent for those over 31 years. Similarly, Vessey *et al* (1986) using as a measure the numbers of previously nulliparous women who had not had either a live or a stillbirth showed a reduction in fertility with age and type of contraceptive used (see Table 5.2). The length of oral contraceptive usage also lengthened the time until the return of fertility (Vessey *et al* 1986), a fact not often reported to couples making their choice of contra-

Table 5.2 The percentage of previously nulliparous women who have not had a live or stillbirth by 48 and 72 months after ceasing contraceptive use (adapted from the work of Vessey *et al* 1986) (nd indicates no data)

Age	Oral contraception		Other methods	
	48 months	72 months	48 months	72 months
25–29	9.1%	nd	7.6%	nd
30–34	17.9%	12.7%	11.5%	10.0%

ceptive method. Because both male and female fertility decreases with age (West 1987), this should be pointed out to couples attending family planning and preconception clinics. In Berryman and Windridge's (1991a) retrospective study of a group of women who had given birth when aged over 40 years, 40 per cent of the primiparous group had sought advice for subfertility compared to only 20 per cent of the multipara.

☐ **Spontaneous abortion**

Stein *et al* (1980) have noted that the risks of spontaneous abortion increase with maternal age whatever the woman's parity, however the authors do point out that this is partly related to the increased chances of chromosomal abnormality with increasing age although the frequency of chromosomally normal abortions also increases. In order to help reduce this risk the woman should, wherever possible, avoid both cigarette smoking before and during pregnancy and drinking alcohol during pregnancy, both of which are known to increase her risk of spontaneous abortion (Plant 1990). In addition smoking during pregnancy produces more frequent intrauterine growth retardation in the older mother (Kuhnert *et al* 1988). (For further information see Plant 1990.) The feasability of preconception advice needs to be questioned since Berryman and Windridge (1991a) showed that 45 per cent of primipara aged over 40 years in their study had not planned the pregnancy and could therefore not have sought any advice.

☐ **Genetic issues**

It has been known for many years that the chances of a child being born handicapped increases with maternal age independent of other risk factors such as socioeconomic status and family history. The abnormalities are mainly chromosomal; congenital defects of unknown aetiology do not increase with maternal age (Baird *et al* 1991).

Screening for fetal abnormality is now available to all older women as part of their antenatal care. It is essential that women themselves are aware of this and also of the necessity of seeking advice early in pregnancy when the widest range of tests including chorion villus sampling is available (Brandenburg *et al* 1991). However, the risk of spontaneous abortion of a normal fetus following chorion villus sampling increases significantly after 36 years of age especially where repeated catheter insertions are required and this must be brought to the attention of couples considering this screening method (Jahoda *et al* 1987).

It has been shown that the use of amniocentesis to screen for fetal abnormality can be reduced by not relying solely on maternal age as an indication. Sheldon and Simpson (1991) and Wald *et al* (1992) have utilised a method of prenatal screening for Down's syndrome which selects those at high risk by using a combination of tests on maternal serum. This so-called 'triple test' includes serum alpha fetoprotein, unconjugated oestriol and human chorionic gonadotrophin estimation. (For further information on this subject see the chapter in this volume by Joanne Whelton on fetal medicine.) Cuckle *et al* (1987) have produced tables which give the woman's risk of carrying a Down's syndrome child in relation to her age, gestation and alpha-fetoprotein level. They have calculated a woman's chances of conceiving a child with Down's syndrome as 1:1572 at age 16, 1:1351 at 25, 1:909 at 30, 1:384 at 35, 1:189 at 38, 1:112 at 40 and 1:37 at 43.

While the existence of screening tests may reduce the chance of the woman giving birth to a handicapped child, the stresses associated with them should not be underestimated. Both the woman and her partner may find the decision about whether or not to have the test (and if so which one), very difficult. Waiting for the results of prenatal tests is stressful and the decision of whether to terminate the pregnancy if the fetus is shown to be abnormal can be extremely painful for both parents. Such stresses can increase the woman's chances of pregnancy and birth complications, such as pregnancy induced hypertension and prolonged labour (Mansfield & Cohn 1986; Mansfield 1988). In Berryman and Windridge's (1991a) survey of the experiences of mothers aged over 40, many voiced fears about possible abnormality although one commented that she wished that the frequency of normal outcome had been stressed to her; this is a potential role for the midwife.

■ Antenatal complications

A number of serious complications of pregnancy have been found to be more common among women aged 35 or over.

□ Hypertensive disease of pregnancy

Chronic hypertension (a blood pressure of more than 140/90 mmHg throughout pregnancy) has been shown to be four times more common among primigravid women aged 35 and over than in primigravidae aged between 20 and 25 (Tuck *et al* 1988). Berkowitz and colleagues (1990) found an increase in hypertensive disease of pregnancy among women aged 35 or more, while Lehmann and Chism's (1987) study of primiparous women in their 40s, attending one North American public hospital, found that they were more likely to develop mild, late onset gestational proteinuric hypertension than either multiparous women of the same age or younger primiparae.

☐ Gestational diabetes

Spellacy *et al* (1986) showed an increase in the frequency of gestational diabetes in women of low parity and normal weight who were aged 40 years or more, when compared with similar women aged 20–30. Specifically, 6.79 per cent of women in the 40 plus age group were found to be suffering from gestational diabetes as compared with 1.69 per cent in the younger age group.

☐ Hydatidiform mole

Bracken (1987), reviewing the incidence and aetiology of this condition, found it to be more common among women of any parity aged 35 and over than in lower age groups. These findings confirmed those of Bagshawe and colleagues (1986) who found that the incidence of the condition among women aged 20–29 was 1 per cent, compared with 1.62 per cent in women aged 35–39 and 2.97 in the 40–44 years age group.

☐ Antepartum haemorrhage

Berkowitz and colleagues (1990) found a greater incidence of antepartum haemorrhage among primiparae over 35 years than in younger age groups. Indeed, antepartum bleeding from any cause was around twice as common in the older women.

■ Labour

Mansfield (1986) in her review found no consistent, methodologically sound, data showing a prolongation of labour. The literature, whilst showing an increase in labour complications and obstetric interventions for older primipara, provides little direct support for the commonly held theories of reduced pelvic mobility. Berkowitz *et al* (1990) in their study of 3917 primiparous women aged over 20 years showed that those aged 30–34 were slightly more likely and those aged 35 or over much more likely to experience labour complications. These included hypertension, fetal distress (although they did not state how this was defined), intrapartum uterine bleeding and a second stage of labour lasting more than two hours.

Cario *et al* (1985) in their study of 127 older primiparae demonstrated that primiparous women aged over 35 years were almost three times more likely than the average for primiparae of all age groups to have a breech presentation (9.4 per cent as opposed to 3.8 per cent), almost twice as likely to require augmentation in labour (53 per cent against 20–37 per cent) and much more likely to have an assisted delivery (28 per cent caesarean section and 35 per cent forceps as compared to 12 per cent caesarean section – see Table 5.3 – and 22–25 per cent forceps). Even when there were no apparent antenatal risk factors, there was a high level of intervention in labour. The authors question whether similar outcomes could have been obtained with less intervention. There was a high rate of low birthweight babies (15 per cent) with two unexplained stillbirths at the start of the third trimester. They state that there is no need, in the absence of other risk factors, to categorise the woman as being at high risk but that this label should still apply to the fetus (Cario *et al* 1985) although there is limited supporting evidence for this recommendation.

Gordon *et al* (1991) have shown an increase in the rate of caesarean section with increasing age of primiparous women with a rate of 33 per cent amongst those over 35 years compared with 24 per cent amongst primipara aged 20–29 years. Where primipara without any complications of pregnancy or labour were considered, those aged over 35 were more than twice as likely to have a caesarean section than were similar women aged 20–29. It was thought by the authors that increasing maternal age influenced the obstetricians to adopt a more 'aggressive' approach (Gordon *et al* 1991) even though research indicates that maternal mortality and morbidity are raised following delivery by caesarean section (Petti 1985; Department of Health 1991). These findings support those by Berkowitz *et al* (1990) and Martel *et al* (1987) (see Table 5.3) with the difference persisting when confounding variables such as the use of epidural anaesthesia, induction of labour and fetal distress were controlled for in the analysis.

Tuck and colleagues' (1988) UK study of primiparous women aged over 35 years showed a caesarean section rate of 27 per cent compared with only 6.6 per cent in those aged 20–25. This includes the high rate of elective caesarean section for women over 35 with a history of subfertility (20.8% of all elective caesareans). The most common reasons for elective caesarean section in the older women were breech presentation – although the value of this is not supported by research (Ingermarsson *et al* 1978) – and maternal age. Fetal distress and failure to progress were the main causes of emergency caesarean sections. Fetal distress was a much more common

Table 5.3 Comparisons of caesarean section rates for older and younger primiparae, with and without complications or a history of subfertility

	Over 35 yrs	20–25 yrs	20–29 yrs	25–35 yrs	All primiparae
Cario *et al* 1985	28%				12%
Martel *et al* 1987	(34+)	(<25)			
	28.2%	13.1%		18.5%	
Tuck *et al* 1988					
– all primiparae	27%	6.6%			
Berkowitz *et al* 1990					
(odds ratios)	1.9		1.0		
Gordon *et al* 1991					
– all primiparae	33%		24%		
– primiparae with no complications of pregnancy/labour	14.3%		6%		

occurrence amongst the older mothers with more of this group having continuous electrical fetal monitoring which in itself increases the risk of operative delivery (MacDonald *et al* 1985). Older women had a longer second stage of labour with a mean of 69 minutes compared with 57 minutes for the younger women (Tuck *et al* 1988). However Friedman and Sachtleben (1965) attribute the longer second stages experienced by older women to higher levels of sedatives given during the first stage of labour. One must question the rationale for their use.

■ Postnatal care

As with most aspects of postnatal care, there is little research into the outcomes for the older first time mother. Jonas and colleagues (1991) have documented that primipara aged over 35 years have longer lengths of hospital stay in the postnatal period for all types of birth when compared with similar women aged 20–29 years. Berryman and Windridge (1991b) reported a difference in the amount of time it took mothers aged over 40 to feel physically 'back to normal' with primipara estimating that it took on average 11.05 months and multipara 7.32 months. The reasons for this are varied and could be due to a different perception of what constitutes normal by the first time mother. In support of this view, whilst the primipara reported more physical changes following the birth there was little difference between the two groups in the amount of 'bother' that these caused. However when the multipara were asked to reflect upon physical symptoms following their first birth, they were less likely to mention these than were the older primipara (Berryman & Windridge 1991b). This makes it appear that the power of physical recovery may slow with increasing age, something for which midwives can prepare mothers in the antenatal period especially if they are planning to return to work quickly or where there are other children in the household. Over 90 per cent of mothers in both groups reported that motherhood when aged over 40 was a very positive experience despite the frequent reports of tiredness with a majority agreeing that the older women had special qualities such as increased patience and understanding. Nearly a third of those surveyed had been mistaken at one time for the child's grandmother which most found amusing (Berryman & Windridge 1991b).

■ Childrearing

Studies have shown that older first time mothers are conscientious parents and in addition their children have lower levels of infant mortality and in particular of sudden infant death (Naeye *et al* 1976) although this could be related to the level of education and socioeconomic conditions. Robinson *et al* (1988) found no overall differences between younger (less than 31 years) and older primipara (over 35 years) in their adjustment to the actual birth of their first child. However the younger group appeared to adapt more quickly to the role of mother (within six months of birth) although this group were less likely to return to work which reduced the degree of adaptation required. The younger women were more likely to see sole responsibility for childcare as their role than the older ones despite the fact that in both groups the women gave the major part of the care (Robinson *et al* 1988). This could give rise to role conflict for the older women especially if they are prevented from resuming activities outside the home.

Higher maternal age has been associated with an increase in measurable intelligence of the children, even taking into account the higher average levels of intelligence for firstborn children (Davie *et al* 1972; Zybert *et al* 1978). The significance of this is probably slight, however, given the strong cultural basis for intelligence tests.

Primiparous women who gave birth over the age of 40 years thought that they experienced more tiredness but that they would be more relaxed in their childrearing than would a woman aged in her 20s (Berryman & Windridge 1991b). In the same survey over half of the older primipara breastfed their infant with an average duration of 6.87 months; this was not compared with a younger group of women.

■ Psychological aspects

Pregnancy is a time of many mixed emotions. Anxiety is common especially in the later weeks together with the occurrence of impatience and mood swings (Chalmers 1982). The older first time mother has the added burden of the common belief that later childbearing is risky for both mother and baby (Mansfield & Cohn 1986) and, as Waters and Wager (1950) stated, this feeling may be exacerbated by more diligent surveillance during pregnancy. In addition the educational level of many of these women and their knowledge about childbearing may increase their stress level if all they read reinforces their worries about older age pregnancy. The existence of books aimed at older first time mothers (Kitzinger 1982; Michelson & Gee 1984) only reinforces the idea that older motherhood is associated with problems.

Price (1977) feels that society itself is prejudiced against older mothers. Berryman and Windridge (1991a) contrast this view to society's attitude to older fatherhood with its proof of sexual activity and virility. The same authors report that women aged over 40 in their survey reported a negative response from family and friends on informing them of the pregnancy. This was despite the fact that over two thirds of the women were happy on finding themselves to be pregnant. About half of the women studied thought that older mothers required 'special treatment or care' and slightly less than this number stated that their doctors had been of the same opinion. Midwives should help to see that this does not become a self-fulfilling prophecy for women in their care. Older primiparous women were more likely to expect pregnancy to be more complicated than if they were aged in their 20s (19 per cent) whereas almost 33 per cent of multipara had experienced an easier pregnancy than previously and only 21.2 per cent one which was more difficult (Berryman and Windridge 1991a). It could be that older primipara attribute any difficulties and problems with pregnancy and child-rearing to their age rather than to it being their first pregnancy.

■ Conclusions

Research in this area seems to show that for the physically well, financially secure and emotionally supported older woman embarking upon her first pregnancy, there is little to worry about. Where the woman has a pre-existing medical condition or a history of subfertility the risk of problems is increased. The woman needs to be made aware of her increased risk of giving birth to a chromosomally abnormal child and given details about screening tests should she so wish. Because these women may worry about putting themselves and their baby at risk due to their age (Mansfield & Cohn 1986), the midwife needs to give time for the woman to voice and discuss her worries.

There is a need for further research into the conduct of labour of these women. The reason for the high rate of caesarean sections – the most frequently found adverse outcome (Mansfield 1986) – with increasing maternal age may be due to worry on the part of obstetricians. Further study is needed, however, to examine progress of labour in the older primigravida. It could be that different parameters will need to be developed for assessing progress in the labours of these women.

There seem to be few major problems in the postnatal period although tiredness and a longer period before the woman feels fully recovered physically have been reported (Berryman & Windridge 1991b). A prospective study with matched groups of older and younger primipara is needed to validate Berryman and Windridge's (1991a, 1991b) retrospective studies.

■ Recommendations for clinical practice in the light of currently available evidence

1. Depending on their past obstetric and medical history women should be given the choice of the type and place of care they wish. For women with no previous problems midwifery care is ideal.

2. The availability of genetic screening tests should be discussed. Care should be taken so as not to cause undue anxiety and to stress how many babies are born normal.

3. Women should be encouraged to talk about their fears and anxieties especially since they will be seen as being at high risk of complications and possibly to have acted foolishly.

4. Older women who are wishing to have a child should be aware of the fact that it may well take longer for them to conceive than it would for younger women.

5. Interventions in labour should only be employed where there is a justifiable reason for their use.

6. Older first time mothers should be made aware that it may well take them longer to return to 'normal' after the birth and that they may experience much tiredness especially if they return to work after a short period of maternity leave.

■ Practice check

● How is the care of older first time mothers 'managed' where you work? Are any generalisations made about age and risk factors? If so, do you agree with them or should they be challenged?

● To what extent is your behaviour towards any woman in your care influenced by preconceived notions about factors such as her age or parity?

- What do you see as the midwife's role in the care of the older first time mother? You may wish to think in particular about helping the woman to make informed choices concerning, for example, prenatal testing, place of birth, care during labour.

- Do you encourage women in your care to discuss their expectations and anxieties about pregnancy, childbirth and parenting?

■ References

Adams M M, Oakley G P, Marks J S 1982 Maternal age and births in the 1980s. Journal of the American Medical Association 247: 493–4

Ales K L, Druzin M L, Santini D L 1990 Impact of maternal age on the outcome of pregnancy. Surgery, Gynecology and Obstetrics 171 (3): 209–216

Baird P A, Sadovnick A D, Yee I M L 1991 Maternal age and birth defects: a population study. Lancet 337: 527–30

Barkan S E, Bracken M B 1987 Delayed childbearing: no evidence for increased risk of low birthweight and preterm delivery. American Journal of Epidemiology 125 (1): 101–9

Berkowitz G S, Skovron M L, Lapinski R H, Berkowitz R L 1990 Delayed childbearing and the outcome of pregnancy. New England Journal of Medicine 322 (10): 659–64

Berryman J C and Windridge K 1991a Having a baby after 40: I. A preliminary investigation of women's experience of pregnancy. Journal of Reproductive and Infant Psychology 9 (1): 3–18

Berryman J C and Windridge K 1991b Having a baby after 40: II. A preliminary investigation of women's experience of motherhood. Journal of Reproductive and Infant Psychology 9 (1): 19–33

Bound J P, Francis B J, Harvey P W 1991 Neural tube defects, maternal cohorts and age: a pointer to aetiology. Archives of Disease in Childhood 66 (10): 1223–6

Bracken M B 1987 Incidence and aetiology of hydatidiform mole: an epidemiological review. British Journal of Obstetrics and Gynaecology 94 (12): 1123–35

Brandenburg H, Van Der Zwan L, Jahoda M G J 1991 Prenatal diagnosis in advanced maternal age. Amniocentesis or CVS, a patient's choice or lack of information? Prenatal Diagnosis 11 (9): 685–90

Bureau of Census 1989 Fertility of American Women: June 1988. Current Population Reports, Series P-20, No 436. US Government Printing Office, Washington DC

Cario G M, Fray R E, Morris N F 1985 The obstetric performance of the elderly primigravida. Journal of Obstetrics and Gynaecology 5: 237–40

Chalmers B 1982 Psychological aspects of pregnancy: Some thought for the eighties. Social Science and Medicine 16: 323–31

Cuckle H S, Wald N J, Thompson S G 1987 Estimating a woman's risk of having a pregnancy associated with Down's syndrome using her age and serum alpha-fetoprotein level. British Journal of Obstetrics and Gynaecology 94 (5): 387–402

Daniels P, Weingarten K 1982 Sooner or later: the timing of parenthood in adult lives. Norton, New York

Davidson E, Fukushima T 1986 The age extremes for reproduction: current implications for policy change. American Journal of Obstetrics and Gynecology 152 (4): 467–71

Davie R, Butler N, Goldstein H 1972 From birth to seven: a report of the National Child Development Study. Longman, London.

Department of Health 1991 Report on confidential enquiries into maternal deaths in the United Kingdom 1985–7. HMSO, London

Edwards R G, Steptoe P C 1983 Current state of in vitro fertilisation and implantation of embryos. Lancet ii: 1265–9

Friedman E, Sachtleben M 1965 Relation of maternal age to the course of labor. American Journal of Obstetrics and Gynecology 9: 915–24

Gaskin I M 1986 Late-bloomers: giving birth after 35. The Birth Gazette 3 (1): 16–17

Gordon D, Milberg J, Daling J, Hickok D 1991 Advanced maternal age as a risk factor for cesarean delivery. Obstetrics and Gynecology 77 (4): 493–7

Harlap S, Shiono P 1980 Alcohol, smoking and incidence of spontaneous abortion in the first and second trimester. Lancet ii: 173–6

Holz K, Cooney C, Marchese T 1989 Outcomes of mature primiparas in an out-of-hospital birth center. Journal of Nurse-Midwifery 34 (4): 185–9

Ingermarsson J, Westgren M, Svenningsen N W 1978 Long term follow-up of pre-term infants and breech presentation delivered by Caesarean section. Lancet ii: 172–5

Jahoda M G J, Pijpers L, Vosters R P L 1987 Role of maternal age in assessment of risk of abortion after prenatal diagnosis during first trimester. British Medical Journal 295: 1237

Jonas O, Chan A, Roder D, Macharper T 1991 Pregnancy outcomes in primigravid women aged 35 years and over in South Australia 1986–88. Medical Journal of Australia 154 (4): 246–9

Kane S H 1967 Advancing age and the primigravida. Obstetrics and Gynecology 29: 409–14

Kirz D S, Dorchester W, Freeman R K 1985 Advanced maternal age: the mature gravida. American Journal of Obstetrics and Gynecology 152 (1): 7–12

Kitzinger S 1982 Birth over thirty. Sheldon Press, London

Kline J, Stein Z A, Susser M W 1977 Smoking: a risk factor for spontaneous abortion. New England Journal of Medicine 297: 793–6

Kline J, Shrout P, Stein Z A 1980 Drinking during pregnancy and spontaneous abortion. Lancet ii: 176–80

Kuhnert B R, Kuhnert P M, Zaelingon T J 1988 Associations between placental cadmium and zinc and age and parity in pregnant women who smoke. Obstetrics and Gynecology 71 (1): 67–70

Lee K, Ferguson R M, Corpuz M 1988 Maternal age and incidence of low birthweight at term: a population study. American Journal of Obstetrics and Gynecology 158 (1): 84–9

Lehmann D, Chism J 1987 Pregnancy outcome in medically complicated and uncomplicated patients age 40 years or over. American Journal of Obstetrics and Gynecology 157 (3): 738–42

MacDonald A, Grant A, Pereira M 1985 The Dublin randomised controlled trial of intrapartum electronic fetal heart rate monitoring. American Journal of Obstetrics and Gynecology 154: 524–39

Mansfield P 1986 Reevaluating the medical risks of late childbearing. Women and Health 11 (2): 37–60

Mansfield P K 1988 Midlife childbearing: strategies for informed decision making. Psychology of Women Quarterly 12 (4): 445–60

Mansfield P K, Cohn M D 1986 Stress and later-life childbearing: important implications for nursing. Maternal and Child Nursing 15 (3): 139–51

Martel M, Wacholder S, Lippman A 1987 Maternal age and primary cesarean section rates: a multivariate analysis. American Journal of Obstetrics and Gynecology 156 (2): 305–8

Michelson J, Gee S 1984 Coming late to motherhood. Thorsons, Wellingborough

Naeye R L 1983 Maternal age, obstetric complications and the outcome of pregnancy. Obstetrics and Gynecology 61: 210–16

Naeye R L, Ladis B, Drage J S 1976 Sudden infant death syndrome: a prospective study. American Journal of Disease in Childhood 130: 1207–10

National Center for Health Statistics 1989 Vital and health statistics. Trends and variations in births to older women, 1970–1976. DHHS Publication No. (PHS) 89-1925 NCHS. Hyattsville, Maryland

Office of Population Censuses and Surveys 1992 Population Trends No. 66, Winter 1991. OPCS, London

Petti D 1985 Maternal mortality and morbidity in cesarean section. Clinical Obstetrics and Gynecology 28: 763–8

Plant M 1990 Maternal alcohol and tobacco use during pregnancy. In Alexander J, Levy V, Roch S (eds) Antenatal Care: A research-based approach (Midwifery Practice, Vol. I) Macmillan, Basingstoke

Poland B J, Miller J R, Jones D C 1977 Reproductive counselling in patients who have had a spontaneous abortion. American Journal of Obstetrics and Gynecology 127: 685–91

Price J 1977 You're not too old to have a baby. Farrar Strauss Giroux, New York

Robinson G E, Garner D M, Gare D J, Crawford B 1987 Psychological adaptation to pregnancy in childless women over 35 years of age. American Journal of Obstetrics and Gynecology 156: 328–33

Robinson G E, Olmsted M, Garner D M, Gare D J 1988 Transition to parenthood in elderly primiparas. Journal of Psychosomatic Obstetrics and Gynaecology 9: 89–101

Sheldon T A, Simpson J 1991 Appraisal of a new scheme for prenatal screening for Down's syndrome. British Medical Journal 302: 1133–6

Spellacy W M, Miller S J, Winegar A 1986 Pregnancy after 40 years of age. Obstetrics and Gynecology 4 (10): 452–4

Stein Z A 1985 A woman's age: childbearing and childrearing. American Journal of Epidemiology 121 (3): 327–42

Stein Z A, Kline J, and Susser E 1980 Maternal age and spontaneous abortion. In Porter I H, Hook E B (eds) Human embryonic and fetal death. Academic Press, New York

Tuck S M, Yudkin P L, Turnbull A C 1988 Pregnancy outcome in elderly primigravidae with and without a history of infertility. British Journal of Obstetrics and Gynaecology   95 (3): 230–7

van Noord-Zaadstra B M, Looman C W N, Alsbach H, Habbema J D F, te Velde E R, Karbaat J 1991 Delaying childbearing: effect of age on fecundity and outcome of pregnancy. British Medical Journal   302: 1361–5

Ventura S 1982 Trends in first births to older mothers 1970–79. National Center for Health Statistics   31 (2): 1–5

Vessey M P, Smith M A, Yeates D 1986 Return of fertility after discontinuation of oral contraceptives: influence of age and parity. British Journal of Family Planning   11: 120–24

Wald N J, Kennard A, Densem W, Cuckle H, Chard T, Butler L 1992 Antenatal maternal serum screening for Down's syndrome: results of a demonstration project. British Medical Journal   305: 391–4

Waters S, Wager H 1950 Pregnancy and labor experiences of elderly primigravidas. American Journal of Obstetrics and Gynecology   59: 296–304

West C P 1987 Age and infertility. British Medical Journal   294: 853–4

Zybert P, Belmont L, Stein Z 1978 Maternal age and children's ability. Perception and Motor Skills   47: 815–18.

■ Suggested further reading

Harker L, Thorpe E 1992 'The last egg in the basket?' Elderly primiparity – a review of findings. Birth   19 (1): 23–30

Mansfield P 1986 Reevaluating the medical risks of late childbearing. Women and Health   11 (2): 37–60

Tuck S M, Yudkin P L, Turnbull A C 1988 Pregnancy outcome in elderly primigravidae with and without a history of subfertility. British Journal of Obstetrics and Gynaecology   95 (3): 230–7

Chapter 6

Couvade – the retaliation of marginalised fathers

Paul Summersgill

This chapter explores the ways in which fathers have been excluded from the processes of pregnancy and childbirth and, arguably, more recently been brought back towards the centre of these activities. Various theories will be put forward which may account for these changes. Throughout, the chapter will focus on the problems created when fathers lack suitable couvade rituals to support them during their partner's pregnancy. It will also explore what can happen when fathers try to gain social recognition for their changed social status by the (re)creation of modern day couvade rituals.

All of the research findings in this chapter are accepted at face value; in a chapter of this size it was considered more important to structure the existing material into a new framework revolving around couvade rather than to attempt any elaborate critique of individual authors. It is hoped that readers will accept this restriction and still find the research discussed useful for their own professional involvement with fathers.

■ **It is assumed that you are already aware of the following:**

- The meaning of the concepts 'power', 'empowerment', 'patriarchy', 'medical control' and 'cascade of intervention';

- That 'reality' is not fixed, but fluid and ever-changing, so that all we ever perceive are 'representations' of behaviour and action as mere 'snapshots' in time;

- That social science can touch on issues which affect individuals very profoundly, so there might be some readers who have intense feelings about fatherhood which may or may not have been opened up to consideration and discussion and which could cause them some distress.

■ Couvade rituals and the loss of fatherhood

Unlike other societies, our culture offers neither institutionalised social support for expectant fathers nor recognition of their importance for creating the baby; all importance is given to the mother not the father (Jordan 1990). By contrast, anthropological studies carried out this century, indicate that many non-Western societies establish important roles for the father to perform during pregnancy and labour (Frazer 1923; Frazer 1925; Dawson 1929; Malinowski 1966). Heggenhougan (1980) suggests that in some such societies fathers are seen as key active participants throughout the birth process. Certainly, some patrilineal Brazilian tribes in South America and others in Montenegro in South East Europe, showed that marginalisation of fathers can be minimised through them being recognised as central to the pregnancy and childbirth process. In these societies fathers were offered considerable social recognition, attention and status through the ritual called 'couvade', which invariably largely excluded the mother (Riviere 1974).

Couvade is taken from the French word 'couver', first used by the anthropologist Tylor (1865) meaning to cover or hatch a nest of eggs or chicks. Riviere (1974) explains that traditionally couvade relates to 'all behaviour associated with childbirth that involves the father giving up his normal routine activities' and following new ritualised behaviour such as social confinement, sexual restraint, avoiding physical labour and certain types of food, and even imitating the birth through mock labour. However, Bettleheim (1955) claims that couvade is ultimately about ensuring that the father is not excluded from the social aspects of parenthood, by guaranteeing that his existence and paternal status are acknowledged in the widest possible context, including if appropriate the adoption of new roles and behaviour patterns.

It was not only fathers in tribal societies who had access to couvade rituals. We have some limited evidence of fairly clearly defined behaviour being expected from fathers in earlier times in our own culture, which went some way towards acknowledging his changed status and power. For instance, Hines (1971) and Bedford and Johnson (1988) have argued that prior to the nineteenth century fathers had a much more clearly defined role than they have today, which formed their couvade ritual. Supposedly, when the baby was due the father knew precisely what was expected of him in terms of carrying firewood, building fires, boiling water and generally assisting in preparing the birth environment.

Unfortunately for fathers, as soon as they were no longer readily available to assist with the birth preparations, midwives began to exclude them from the birth process (Hines 1971). Hines considers that this inability of the father to perform the anticipated and beneficial couvade rituals surrounding childbirth was due to the increased separation of workplace and home, physically taking the father away from his partner. Alternatively, the location of birth shifted from home to hospital where obstetricians and midwives believed that *they* should provide all that the mother would need. In this way, fathers lost their links with the very couvade behaviours which had previously brought them *some* public acknowledgement and recognition as fathers; fatherhood entailing public and private ritual largely evaporated.

One of the more serious consequences of these changes is that, whilst motherhood has long been recognised as a meaningful social concept, fatherhood has barely been acknowledged beyond its biological dimension of procreating a child (David 1985). In the words of Homans (1985), regrettably 'fatherhood is rarely seen to be as defining of men as motherhood seems to be of women'. This is reflected in the masses of material written about mothers and motherhood, while only in the last decade or so have fathers and fatherhood been rediscovered by social scientists as fathers have tried to establish new couvade rituals to lend credence to their social – as opposed to biological – existence (Richards 1981; Hanson & Bozett 1985; Lewis & Salt 1986; Lewis & O'Brien 1987). The limited amounts of literature about fatherhood that do exist remain problematic moreover, because they have tended to focus on the clinical contexts in which fathers can assist with labour and delivery, largely ignoring other social dimensions surrounding pregnancy and birth, such as fathers' own needs for couvade.

The overall public indication given to and reluctantly adopted by fathers was that they should only play peripheral or background roles and be prepared to accept merely token acknowledgement of their existence by midwives (Richman & Goldthorp 1978). In clinical practice this invariably resulted in hospital staff dismissing fathers or treating them as children or 'semi-comical' characters, giving them 'pretend' birth roles such as being allowed to cut the cord (Barbour 1986). Typically, the father's presence on the labour ward was only tolerated by the health care team on the grounds of his ability to act as an unpaid carer, particularly during times of staff shortages and economic crises (Keirse 1989).

Similarly, in the domestic realm, if the social context was mentioned at all for fathers, it was largely in playing a financially and emotionally supportive role for their partners (Richards 1981), rather than offering any advice about their own status and power needs as a father; appropriate couvade rituals as such were never mentioned.

☐ **The rise of the marginalised father**

Kitzinger (1980) maintains that this, not surprisingly, complicated the transition to fatherhood, making many fathers feel marginalised, isolated, resentful and guilty. It also meant that fathers emerged in the eyes of society as poorly qualified and badly equipped to play anything more than a minor role in childbirth and later infant care.

Many marginalised fathers being denied any significant role to play actually began to believe that they were unnecessary participants throughout pregnancy, labour and childbirth (Rapoport & Rapoport 1977). Certainly part of this assessment of the marginalised father's role was based on the assumption that men are not especially interested in the process of childbirth (Bedford & Johnson 1988). Indeed, this became something of a self-fulfilling prophecy when some fathers underlined their acceptance of this medical assessment of their marginalised status and role by developing subcultural beliefs that their possible involvement with the pregnancy would threaten their masculinity and virility. Such 'self-inflicted' marginalisation involved fathers preferring to hand over complete control to 'experts' in an attempt to sustain their limited status (Kitzinger 1980). Romalis (1981) endorses this idea further by asserting that there is a widespread belief amongst men in many cultures that once they have played the important and irreplaceable role of 'planting the seed', their duties are largely completed at least until after the birth.

☐ **Lack of couvade rituals and fathers' 'pregnancy careers'**

Unlike expectant mothers who have their new status, position and role clarified in various social locations, no such changes are made obvious to marginalised expectant fathers (Richman and Goldthorp 1978). Expectant mothers throughout their pregnancies have their maternity careers endorsed commercially, socially and medically, but no such provision is made for men in recognition of their role and status as fathers (despite the existence of birth registration which keeps the father's changed identity invisible to all but a few administrators). Moran-Ellis (1989) claims that the father's role has been marginalised in that it has never been made clear in either a professional or statutory sense, merely remaining undefined and voluntary for the most part. As if to undermine the father still further, Jordan (1990) suggests that coping with a marginalised role often has to be handled without the benefit of institutionalised social support, like couvade.

Undoubtedly, becoming a father can be a major life crisis for many men, and can be just as stressful for the father as the transition to motherhood is for the woman (Kitzinger 1983). Lacking couvade rituals to guide them through the pregnancy and birth, Richman (1982) has argued that fathers develop what can be termed a 'pregnancy career' in the sense that the duration of the pregnancy can profoundly affect other aspects of their lives. Obviously pregnancy careers can take many forms and directions and involve differing degrees of personal crisis. Nevertheless, there are some generalisations that can be made about the possibility of health and social problems arising for fathers trying to cope with their partner's pregnancy (Perkins 1980; Romalis 1981; Clinton 1987; Benvenuti *et al* 1989; Bothamley 1990).

Lacking a well developed and significant role or status both antenatally and postnatally, and without appropriate rituals to support them, many fathers develop what Romalis (1981) refers to as their own 'pregnancy symptomatology'. This consists of a variety of sometimes conflicting symptoms including feelings of nausea, headache, toothache, depression, irritability, fatigue, insomnia, loss of appetite and weight gain (Kupferer 1965; Newman 1966; Fawcett & York 1986; Strickland 1987). Clinton (1986) argues that we should regard these symptoms as constituting an embryonic form of couvade because they are an attempt by the father to get other people to recognise the causes of his problems, namely a lack of social recognition for his changed role and status.

Trethowan and Conlan's (1965) research was amongst the earliest evidence based on sound methodology to demonstrate that expectant fathers do indeed experience an increase in specific ailments during their partner's pregnancy, particularly during the third and ninth months. Surprisingly, Richman and Goldthorp (1978) and Romalis (1981) claim that neither most fathers nor their GPs would recognise the connection between the father's lack of social status and role during pregnancy and these symptoms.

In parallel with their own pregnancy symptomatology, Parke (1982) reports that fathers are often, also, far more aware of their partner's symptoms than are the mothers themselves. This 'adopted' pregnancy symptomatology could be regarded as a supplementary form of couvade behaviour used by the father to confirm publicly his changed status. An alternative explanation developed from Bedford and Johnson (1988) indicates that fathers not only have to cope with their own transition to fatherhood, but also that of their partner to motherhood. One way of coping with the partner's transition to motherhood might be to become engrossed in the mother's health problems, including grieving with her if a stillbirth occurs (Healy 1990).

Research based on the work of family therapists such as Rapoport and Rapoport (1977) indicates that, whilst marginalised fathers may well be proud and overjoyed by the birth of their babies, lacking appropriate couvade rituals they are also very uncertain about their futures and the responsibilities which becoming a father brings (Trethowan & Conlan 1965; Kitzinger 1983; Clinton 1987). For some marginalised fathers, the difficulty they face in coping with changed interpersonal and sexual relations with their partners can be of considerable importance (Gill 1989). Unavailability of suitable couvade rituals focusing upon their needs might lead to fathers becoming jealous of the attention the mother receives during pregnancy and motherhood, or of the mother's preoccupation with the baby rather than her partner. In this way couvade rituals, or the lack of them, can take on great significance because of the enormous conflict which can potentially occur in relationships (Roopnarine & Miller 1985).

Many other important social problems can occur because fathers lack access to couvade rituals which would serve to support them if these problems developed. Commonly, marginalised fathers who want to support their partners as much as they can during pregnancy become very concerned about the loss of income which their presence at the antenatal clinic or antenatal class might entail (Bothamley 1990). Yet, at the same time, fathers might want to learn how to look after their babies in order to help overcome feelings of being second rate carers and thus feel pressurised to attend in spite of this difficulty (Thompson 1982; Kitzinger 1983).

Similar financial difficulties might also be encountered by fathers in attending the labour and birth (Richman & Goldthorp 1978). Once the baby is born, if fathers are in paid work outside the home they can find it difficult to spend the amount of time they would ideally wish to spend with their newborn and partner (Bothamley 1990). Also, many fathers have a need for knowledge about general aspects of parenting after the baby is born, rather than information which simply concentrates on preparation for birth (Thompson 1982). Although many fathers make enthusiastic comments about the relevance and usefulness of antenatal classes, and are usually made to feel welcome by the midwifery team on the labour ward by being offered information and encouragement to help reduce their feelings of inadequacy, Pratt (1990) suggests there still remains the fundamental problem that insufficient attention is paid to fathers at all stages of the pregnancy and labour, and no suitable couvade activities are offered to them.

□ **Lack of couvade rituals and hospitalisation**

Richman (1982) has argued that many fathers feel that the processes of admitting their partners to hospital serves further to marginalise themselves, by underlining their powerlessness compared with the extensive 'medical' power and control over birth. It also indicates fathers' need for some supportive rituals to help them cope with the experience of hospitalisation. Despite an absence of couvade activities, Moran-Ellis (1989) asserts that many fathers still manage to feel in control of their role in relation to the pregnancy until the decision is made to transfer the mother to hospital, at which point the father (and mother) are subject to the control and authority of 'medical' staff. Moreover, this loss of control can occur even before the father physically enters the hospital building because the decision to admit the mother is often influenced by 'expert' knowledge provided in consultation with hospital staff over the telephone.

Whilst mothers may be reasonably well prepared to enter the hospital environment to give birth as a result of their participation at antenatal classes, fathers are less likely to be so. This could further amplify their marginalised status and demonstrates the need for suitable preparation to help them through this difficult stage. Some men, unprepared by couvade ritual, experience 'entrance trauma' once in hospital, especially when they are there for the birth of their first child. These experiences manifest themselves in the father's perception of the hospital as a culturally alien environment, where he encounters a mass of nameless, faceless experts using a 'foreign' medical language, together with a barrage of technological gadgets (Inch 1989). Such problems as having their partners taken away from them in the reception area, being largely ignored by midwives after the initial introductions and being made to feel a stranger or an outsider in what is seen by midwives to be only 'women's business', were common complaints (Thompson 1982). Equally perplexing are the unclarified and limited role and rights his marginalised status gives a father.

Berry (1988) expresses concern that for many men lacking suitable couvade ritual preparation, labour becomes a time of great stress in which they try to hide their feelings and worry about their uselessness in assisting their partners through the birth. The extent of fathers' marginalised role and status can be summarised in the expectation of many midwives that fathers should co-operate by keeping a very low profile, staying well out of the way of all decision making and action during the childbirth process (Keirse 1989).

☐ **Lack of couvade post delivery**

Fathers also need to develop couvade coping skills and appropriate social support *after* their baby has been born, yet ironically, this does not often happen. For instance, after the birth has occurred, fathers are sometimes further excluded from contact with their partners and babies (Inch 1989). At what is probably a momentous moment in both partners' lives (Jackson 1984), the father is expected by the midwifery team to conform to their routines and return home, in symbolic and practical terms temporarily abandoning both mother and baby. This separation might be seen by both partners as inappropriate since they might require considerable amounts of time together after the birth to talk about and share the birth experience and the baby. Inch (1989) has argued that for some fathers this period when they return home from hospital, together with limited visiting hours, can become a time of great loneliness and depression. Moreover, for many fathers this time away from partners is regarded as time wasted when they could be learning childcare skills as part of their couvade activities, merely serving to reinforce that it is the mothers who have these skills, knowledge and expertise, leaving the father feeling inadequate once more (Feltz 1986). Proof that couvade rituals can be of benefit to fathers is provided by Swedish evidence (Lind 1974), which suggests that involving fathers in acquiring childcare skills in hospital can lead to them feeling less disempowered and prepared to take a more active and prolonged involvement in childcare at home.

■ Responses to marginalisation

The offering of trivial roles and status to marginalised fathers was challenged by feminists such as Kitzinger (1980). They argued that many fathers were increasingly not marginalised and were empowering themselves by becoming actively involved in many aspects of domestic life, including the care of their pregnant partners; in a very real sense seeking out their own couvade rituals.

Romalis (1981) proposed that this can also be explained by changes in the strict division of domestic labour in families. He claims that relationships between partners (and their children) have become increasingly democratic, egalitarian and symmetrical. Although many feminists would doubt the extent of these changes, where they have occurred they represent an eroding of traditional patriarchal values and behaviour (Oakley 1974; Edgell 1980; Boulton 1983; Allan 1985). Because of men's relatively new gender roles, involving a more child centred approach to family life combined with their increased participation in domestic labour, men are now choosing to be present at the birth of their babies where previously they would have remained relative outsiders to the process (Alibhai 1988). Recognising the growing awareness that parenthood should not be about marginalisation of one partner at the expense of the other, but about the involvement of both partners, the plea by McKee (1980) for the father's role 'to be made more coherent, explicit and accepted', summed up the growing feeling that fathers needed to expand their developing couvade rituals.

☐ The rise of the progressive father

Consequently, from a tendency which began in the 1970s (Cronenwett & Newmark 1974), slowly acknowledging the importance of fatherhood during pregnancy and labour, hospital policy began to try to integrate fathers into the process (Brown 1982; Barbour 1990). This was so fundamental and widespread a change that, by the 1980s, hospitals were apparently no longer marginalising fathers, but instead both permitting and encouraging all fathers to be present during childbirth, so that they might actively assist with the emotional and psychological dimensions of their partner's labour (Keirse 1989). In this way, midwives could be regarded as helping to create and sustain new couvade rituals for fathers in hospital, by giving them tasks to perform as well as providing greater public acknowledgement of their importance during childbirth. These adjustments went some way towards enabling marginalised fathers to play a significant role as 'new men', so much so that Romalis (1981) suggested that they should more accurately be referred to as 'progressive' fathers. However, according to May (1982) it has to be remembered that it is largely the pregnant woman who determines the extent of the father's involvement during childbearing, so fathers might still remain partially marginalised in spite of some improvements in organisational policy.

☐ Couvade 'solutions' to marginalisation

Some progressive fathers, previously marginalised by their lack of status and role antenatally, have attempted to introduce their own modern day couvade rituals.

In terms of their social and work roles, fatherhood is used by some fathers as an opportunity for changes in behaviour and restructuring of their social identities. Some fathers, anticipating the extra costs involved when the baby arrives, spend more time at work to earn extra cash or take on a more responsible approach to work (Dodendorf 1981; Parke 1982). Some fathers might try to physically underline their changed social status and responsibility by altering their appearance, perhaps by growing a moustache (Bittman & Zalk 1978). On the domestic front, couvade might consist of completing jobs around the home (especially preparing the baby's room) and of taking a more active part in looking after any other children (Benvenuti *et al* 1989).

In terms of sexual behaviour, couvade often consists of deliberately abstaining from sexual intercourse with their partner, a very important symbolic gesture which underlines the immense value of both the partner and the baby for the father. This is often seen by fathers to be one of their main contributions to a successful birth outcome, especially if a previous pregnancy resulted in a miscarriage. It also reflects and lends support to a widespread fear that both partners might have that intercourse is potentially damaging to the baby's health (Lumley & Astbury 1989).

Progressive fathers will have also spent considerable amounts of time preparing themselves for the pregnancy and birth, especially in acquiring skills of self-confidence and assertiveness (Romalis 1981). Moran-Ellis (1989) provides examples of the kinds of couvade activities middle class fathers expect to be involved with during pregnancy and labour. For instance, fathers expect to acquire technical knowledge about childbirth which will assist them in helping their partners make decisions about labour options. On the labour ward fathers expect to be allowed to acquire information from 'medical' staff which can then be used by themselves and their partners to decide upon appropriate methods of pain control. Fathers are also empowered by playing the role of 'technology watcher', using the fetal monitoring equipment to predict contraction patterns for partners, or in following the baby's progress. (Currently no health care team would ever rely entirely on the father to perform this task however.)

Besides being in a commanding position as companion, witness and comforter for their partners, Moran-Ellis (1989) offers evidence of fathers empowering themselves through controlling access to pain relief for their partners, and by questioning and doubting the need for such relief. Fathers also extend their control by acting as gatekeepers, taking 'responsibility for maintaining or achieving the goals the couple ... set before labour had started', such as avoiding an epidural or giving birth in a certain position.

☐ **The 'rejection' of progressive fathers**

Clearly, whilst this might be beneficial to the father, midwives and mothers could have very mixed feelings about the partner's growing involvement in decisions which profoundly affect the mother. Nevertheless, the route to a successful birth experience for many progressive fathers is to acquire full 'medical' information on which they and their partners can base any decisions and to have an equal relationship with the health care team. If this is valid and feasible, we can expect ever-increasing numbers of men to be participating in all aspects and stages of their partner's childbirth and wanting to become more involved than they did in the past (Bothamley 1990).

Whilst all of these new couvade rituals might have benefits for the father, there is an undoubted downside to these activities as far as some women are concerned; the progressive father's presence does not automatically bring about a significant contribution to a positive birth experience for the mother (Di Renzo *et al* 1981; Odent 1984). Even though there are various pieces of research (Goldthorp & Richman 1974; Richman & Goldthorp 1978; Niven 1985; Bothamley 1990) which show that the father's presence during the birth process can have beneficial effects on the quality of the mother's labour experiences, such as the reduced perception of pain during labour (Henneborn & Cogan 1975) and a lessened need for medication, this is by no means a universal feature.

Undoubtedly, for some women the partner's presence and couvade activities might actually be evaluated as unhelpful, the mothers preferring to be alone without having to worry about upsetting their partners by the pain childbirth can include. Odent (1984) goes so far as to claim that the father's presence during childbirth can be detrimental in that it actually slows down labour. This can be understood by appreciating that mothers need to concentrate during labour and an anxious father who talks too much or who is overly fearful might distract his partner. Additionally, some fathers might be overprotective or very possessive of the mothers and, instead of calming them, only manage to overstimulate their partners through constant massaging or holding. These kinds of factors can prevent the mother from expressing her own instinctive behaviour.

Additional research by Di Renzo *et al* (1981) endorses the viewpoint that mothers might well be better off without fathers during childbearing. Two thirds of Di Renzo's Italian research sample indicated that they would have preferred someone other than their partner with them during labour.

This might be due to major tensions in the couple's relationship which make it difficult for either partner to give or receive practical and emotional support during labour. For some women it might be preferable to emphasise their right to choose whom they want with them during labour, and not to over emphasise the seemingly automatic right of the father to be present (O'Driscoll & Meager 1980).

Certainly, Romito (1986) is not entirely convinced about the need to empower fathers by providing them with new couvade activities which help to move them away from their earlier marginalised role and status. As illustrated above, it has to be questioned whether for control to be held by fathers is really in the mothers' best interests. In fact, who does benefit apart from the fathers from their having gained new couvade rituals and a more progressive role? For Romito, even if fathers are allowed to be more actively involved with labour, thereby giving both partners the impression that the maternity hospital routines have been humanised, full approval for the carrying out of couvade activities is only allowed with the approval of the 'medical' staff, who as ever, still hold the reins of real power and control of the birth situation.

Slowly, progressive fathers have begun to realise that they can only really carry out couvade rituals within a hospital context by obtaining the sanction of the health care team. Unfortunately, their endless pursuit of the perfect couvade ritual within the hospital has helped to create what is potentially a much more dangerous kind of partner for the mother – defined as a 'pregnancy policeman' by Bradley, an American obstetrician, over a quarter of a century ago.

☐ **Reactionary fathers: couvade and medical control**

Controversially, what Bradley (1965) advocated was a method of ensuring that the expectant mother behaved as the health care team saw fit, and not necessarily offering what either the mother or father felt they needed. This high degree of 'medical' control over the birth would be achieved because the father would be provided with more social recognition of his importance during labour and birth by the health care team, in return for his absolute 'co-operation' and support for the clinical procedures on offer to his partner. By this means, the mother's opportunities for doubt or criticism of what she received would be restricted and make life much easier for the professionals.

To what extent this American idea was picked up and developed elsewhere during the 1960s is uncertain, but by the 1980s it was becoming apparent that an understanding and explanation of the father's role during pregnancy and childbirth in any clinical setting had to take into account his social control function as 'policeman'.

Some limited acknowledgement of the existence of Bradley's 'pregnancy policemen' (who would now more appropriately be regarded as 'reaction-ary' fathers) has been provided by Romalis (1981) and Romito (1986). They suggest that the health care team have only been prepared to bring fathers into the processes of pregnancy and childbirth as part of a strategy to increase and maintain 'medical' control over childbearing women. The health care team recognised fathers' needs for even more pronounced couvade rituals in hospital and decided to use this desire for their clinical advantage. In agreeing to bring fathers more directly into the processes of childbearing, the health care team demanded as their price that fathers should agree to establish a 'power bond' with them, designed to reinforce the domination of 'experts' and the superiority of obstetric and midwifery opinion over lay needs.

As a temporary co-opted member of the health care team assisting the woman, reactionary fathers are now expected to agree with the obstetrician and midwives' definition and assessment of the birth situation and to reject any contrary requests from the mother for different treatment as mere infantile whims. In essence, then, the relationship between the father and the health care team might strengthen and support his couvade activities, but actually lead to more rather than less 'medical' intervention for the mother (National Institutes of Health 1981; Copstick *et al* 1986). Romalis (1981) urges us to believe that most expectant fathers can cope with this deceit and betrayal of their partners by rationalising it as being fundamentally beneficial to both mother and child. For example, if a medical intervention (such as induction of labour) is suggested by the obstetric team, the suggestion may be regarded by the father as being based upon scientific and technical knowledge held only by obstetricians (Arney 1982), and therefore to be followed without question. So, by sharing the burden of responsibility for a safe birth with the health care team, the expectant father invariably comes to share their conventional view of pregnant women as in need of management and 'medical' intervention – something most fathers are only too happy to leave in the 'safe' hands of their partner's health care team. The problem, from the woman's point of view, with this situation is that, along with the father's increased couvade status, she loses a potential ally in her male partner and gains a traitor instead (Alibhai 1988). Although largely influenced by North American childbearing practice, this line of argument is sufficiently worrying to make it fundamentally worth examining by midwives and obstetricians in the United Kingdom when assessing their own rationale for involving fathers during childbirth.

Finally, additional support for the increasing existence of reactionary fathers comes from Rothman (1982) who provides the example of fathers being encouraged by obstetricians to act as their partner's 'labour coach', as suggested by the French Lamaze technique. Unfortunately, Rothman regards the reason for using the technique as being slightly sinister inasmuch, once again, that it is more about maintaining obstetric and midwifery dominance on the labour ward than offering a more positive birth experience.

Rothman's argument is that the technique has the effect of making the mother non-complaining, obedient and co-operative with the health care team. Essentially, fathers are on hand in the labour ward to ensure that their partners constantly engage in the procedures of the technique, thereby keeping the woman quiet, uncomplaining and relatively passive by giving her a task to do. Once again, fathers have their social status and purpose endorsed publicly with these additional couvade activities, but are seen by Rothman as being duped into assisting with a medicalised birth by playing a reactionary patriarchal role in 'supervising' labour and childbirth.

At the end of the day, the pursuit and extension of meaningful couvade rituals by fathers has arguably served no one's needs – certainly not the mother's, probably not the father's and, quite possibly, not those of the health care team either.

■ Conclusions

This chapter has attempted to do a number of things. It has explored the problematic nature of fatherhood, focusing especially upon fathers' experiences during pregnancy and childbirth. It has related fathers' behaviour to their attempts to gain some social recognition for their new position as fathers through the development and application of the ritual known as couvade. Clearly, it is not the case that all experiences of fatherhood are similar – there is undoubtedly a wide variation of individual experiences – but this chapter has argued for the existence of three key types of fatherhood which are linked to different amounts of involvement in couvade ritual.

A common assumption suggests that 'normal' fatherhood is uncomplicated and simply about fathers acting as their partner's advocate, helping mothers in a variety of ways during pregnancy and childbirth, in some kind of universally altruistic way. This chapter has suggested that the picture is far more complicated and that different types of behaviour from fathers depends upon their search for new couvade activities to play which endorse their changed social status, offering them support and recognition. Specifically, it has been suggested that particular forms of fatherhood have to be understood as the outcome of complex interactions between fathers, mothers and the health care team, each having various degrees of influence on how the father should behave in what they see as an 'appropriate' way.

It has been proposed that, although historically and in other cultures fathers knew what was expected of them because of explicit couvade rituals setting out their position, until recent years in the West very few couvade rituals have been available to help structure fathers' status and role. Consequently, lacking a clearly defined purpose, many fathers were often left stranded on the very periphery of the birth process by midwives; such fathers have been referred to here as marginalised fathers. It has been suggested that all of this changed during the 1970s when, dissatisfied with their marginalised status, many fathers tried to forge new couvade rituals for themselves, both before and during childbirth. What emerged were progressive fathers, for whom a significant part of their couvade was a decision to play a very active role in all aspects of the pregnancy and labour. It was the emergence of this type of 'new' father which gave the impression that fathers were automatically useful advocates for their partners, apparently only acting in the interests of the mother.

There is concern, however, that out of a genuine desire by fathers to assist their partners in whatever supportive role they can, may come a 'darker' type of father. This third type of father, the reactionary father, has been shown to be much more concerned with establishing and maintaining his needs and concerns than genuinely helping his partner to fulfil hers. This has been shown to represent the most threatening of all couvade rituals adopted by fathers, since it involves the father effectively joining forces with the health care team and supporting whatever recommendations they decide are appropriate for the mother, irrespective of the mother's own wishes.

■ Recommendations for clinical practice in the light of currently available evidence

1. Of paramount importance is the need to carry out further research to investigate the existence of the three 'types' of father identified in this chapter, especially the reactionary father or 'pregnancy policeman'.

2. It is vital that all members of the midwifery team recognise and work with the process of fatherhood. Emphasis should be placed not just on the clinical contexts of fatherhood, but also on its wider social contexts.

3. Recognition should be given to the existence of pregnancy careers for fathers, often involving elaborate couvade rituals and behaviour changes. The midwifery team need to decide to what extent and why they are prepared to support these rituals and behaviour, and to consider the implications of this for a successful or less successful birth outcome. Additional social support might be needed for fathers in helping them to adjust to their new role and status.

4. The midwifery team needs to acknowledge the father's pregnancy symptomatology when discussing family health problems. Ways and means have to be found to assist fathers in either avoiding or coping with the assorted health and social problems of pregnancy.

5. Decisions have to be made by the midwifery team about whether and

why they want to involve fathers significantly during pregnancy and labour. It has to be acknowledged that certain 'types' of fatherhood might be more advantageous to the father than to the mother. Balances of power which exist between the midwifery team and the parents need investigation and where necessary adjustment.

6. Attitudes and approaches of the midwifery team to the father need elaborate investigation to ensure that a positive birth experience is offered for him too. It cannot be assumed that any of the three 'types' of fatherhood described in this chapter are acceptable for any of the parties involved. A new type of fatherhood is needed which does not exclude fathers, over empower them at the expense of mothers, or involve them 'selling out' by totally integrating themselves into the health care team.

7. Consideration might be given to encouraging more home births in low risk circumstances, partly as a way of producing new roles and status for fathers which does not encroach on the mother's power and significance, nor reinforce the justification for medically controlled births, but which moves towards a balance of power, status and role between the partners.

8. The midwifery team must not assume that mothers want their partners with them during childbirth. Time must be spent with the mother finding out who she really wants with her. Ways must be found of both implementing her request and of defusing the marital conflict which might arise if the father's presence is not requested by her.

■ Practice check

- Can you recognise couvade symptoms in fathers? How do you respond to such behaviour?

- How can you help fathers adjust to fatherhood?

- Do you encourage fathers to take part in antenatal and postnatal classes?

- How do you help to make fatherhood significant for fathers on the labour ward?

- How can you set about identifying and responding to the differing needs and expectations of fathers on the labour ward?

- How did you handle your last (if any) disagreement with a father? How successful was the outcome and what changes in the process might you need to make in future?

■ References

Alibhai Y 1988 Trouble and strife. New Statesman and Society   1 (24): 22–3

Allan G 1985 Family life: domestic roles and social organization. Blackwell, London

Arney W R 1982 Power and the profession of obstetrics. University of Chicago Press, Chicago

Backwell J 1977 Husband in the labour ward. Midwives Chronicle   90–91: 270–2

Barbour R S 1986 Being there: fathers on the labour ward. Paper presented at the British Sociological Association Medical Sociology Conference, York, 26–28 September

Barbour R S 1990 Fathers: the emergence of a new consumer group. In Garcia J, Kilpatrick R, Richards M (eds) The politics of maternity care. Clarendon Press, Oxford

Bedford V A, Johnson N 1988 The role of the father. Midwifery   4: 190–5

Benvenuti P, Marchetti G, Tozzi G, Pazzagli A 1989 Psychological and psychopathological problems of fatherhood. Journal of Psychosomatic Obstetrics and Gynaecology Supplement   10: 35–41

Bittman S, Zalk S 1978 Expectant Fathers. Hawthorn Books, New York

Berry L M 1988 Realistic expectations of the labour coach. Journal of Obstetric, Gynecologic and Neonatal Nursing 17   (5): 354–5

Bettleheim B 1955 Symbolic wounds: puberty rites and the envious male. Thames and Hudson, London

Bothamley J 1990 Are fathers getting a fair deal? Nursing Times   86 (36): 68–9

Boulton M G 1983 On being a mother. Tavistock Publications, London

Bradley R 1965 Husband-coached childbirth. Harper and Row, New York

Brown A 1982 Fathers in the labour ward: medical and lay accounts. In McKee L, O'Brien M (eds) The father figure. Tavistock Publications, London

Clinton J 1987 Physical and emotional responses of expectant fathers throughout pregnancy and the early postpartum period. International Journal of Nursing Studies   24 (1): 59–68

Clinton J F 1986 Expectant fathers at risk of couvade. Nursing Research   35 (5): 290–95

Copstick S M, Taylor K E, Hayes R, Morris N 1986 Partner support and the use of coping behaviour in labour. Journal of Psychosomatic Research   30: 497–503

Cronenwett L R, Newmark L L 1974 Fathers' responses to childbirth. Nursing Research   23 (3): 210–17

David M 1985 Motherhood and social policy – a matter of education? Critical Social Policy   12: 28–43

Dawson W 1929 The custom of couvade. University Press, Manchester

Di Renzo G C, Bruni R, Villoti C, Bimi P, Boselli S, Ricchi A, Vecchi S, Montanari G D 1981 Clima Psicologico in Sala Parto, Gli Ospedali della Vita   27, 28, 29 (Supplement: 65–84)

Edgell S 1980 Middle-class couples. Allen Lane, London

Entwistle D R, Doering S G 1981 The first birth. Johns Hopkins University Press, Baltimore

Dodendorf D 1981 Expectant fatherhood and first pregnancy. The Journal of Family Practice   13 (5): 744–51

Fawcett J, York R 1986 Spouses' physical and psychological symptoms during pregnancy and postpartum. Nursing Research 35 (3): 144–8

Feltz V 1986 First-time fathers. Parents (September): 71–72, 77

Frazer J G 1923 Folk-lore in the Old Testament. Macmillan, London

Frazer J G 1925 The Golden Bough – a study in magic and religion. Macmillan, London

Gill L 1989 No place for a man. The Times June 9

Goldthorp W O, Richman J 1974 Reorganization of the maternity services – a comment on domiciliary confinements in view of the experience of the hospital strike, 1973. Midwife, Health Visitor and Community Nurse 10: 265–71

Hanson S M H, Bozett F W 1986 Dimensions of fatherhood. Sage, Beverly Hills

Healy P 1990 Where fathers can cry, too. The Independent April 2: 14

Heggenhougen M 1980 Father and childbirth: an anthropological perspective. Journal of Nurse Midwifery 25 (6): 21–5

Henneborn W J, Cogan R 1975 The effect of husband participation on reported and probability of medication during labour and birth. Journal of Reproductive and Infant Psychology 3: 45–53

Hines J D 1971 Father – the forgotten man. Nursing Forum 10 (2): 176–200

Homans H (ed) 1985 The sexual politics of reproduction. Gower, Aldershot: 124

Inch S 1989 Birthrights – a parents' guide to modern childbirth, 2nd edn. Green Print, London

Jackson S 1984 Becoming a father. Nursery World July 5th: 6–7

Jordan P L 1990 Laboring for relevance: expectant and new fatherhood. Nursing Research 39: 11–16

Keirse M J N C 1989 Social and professional support during childbirth. In Chalmers I, Enkin M, Keirse M (eds) Effective Care in Pregnancy and Childbirth, Vol 2: 805–814. Oxford University Press, Oxford

Kitzinger S 1980 Pregnancy and childbirth. Michael Joseph, London

Kitzinger S 1983 Birth over thirty. Sheldon Press, London

Kupferer H 1965 Couvade: ritual or real illness? American Anthropologist 67: 99–102

Lewis C, O'Brien M 1987 Reassessing fatherhood. Sage Publications, London

Lewis R A, Salt R E 1986 Men in families. Sage, Beverly Hills

Lind J 1974 Observations after delivery of communications between mother, infant and father. International Congress of Paediatrics, October 1974, Buenos Aires

Lumley J, Astbury J 1989 Advice for pregnancy. In Chalmers I, Enkin M, Keirse M (eds) Effective Care in Pregnancy and Childbirth, Vol 1: 237–54. Oxford University Press, Oxford

Malinowski B 1966 The father in primitive psychology. Norton Library, New York

May K A 1982 Three phases of father involvement in pregnancy. Nursing Research 31 (6): 337–42

May K A, Perrin S P 1985 Prelude: pregnancy and birth. In Hanson S M H, Bozett F W (eds) Dimensions of fatherhood. Beverly Hills

McKee L 1980 Fathers and childbirth: just hold my hand. Health Visitor 53 (9): 368–72

McKee L, O'Brien M 1982 The father figure. Tavistock, London

Moran-Ellis 1989 The role of the father in childbirth. Midwife, Health Visitor and Community Nurse   25 (7): 284–8

National Institutes of Health 1981 Cesarean childbirth. Report of a consensus development conference, NIH Publication No. 82-2067. US Department of Health and Human Services. Public Health Service. National Institutes of Health, Bethesda

Newman L 1966 The couvade: a reply to Kupferer. American Anthropologist   68: 153–6

Niven C 1985 How useful is the presence of the husband at childbirth? Journal of Reproductive and Infant Psychology   3: 45–53

Oakley A 1974 Housewife. Allen Lane, London

Odent M 1984 Birth reborn. Souvenir Press, London

O'Driscoll K, Meager D 1980 Active management of labour. W B Saunders, London

Parke R D 1982 Fathering the developing child. Fontana, Glasgow

Perkins E R 1980 Men of the labour ward. Levenhulme Health Education Project, Occasional Paper No. 22. University of Nottingham

Pratt D 1990 The partner's role in pregnancy. Nursing   4 (9): 23–4

Rapoport R, Rapoport R 1977 Fathers, mothers and others. Routledge, London

Richards M 1981 And father came too. Nursing Mirror   153 (17): viii–xi

Richman J, Goldthorp W O 1978 Fatherhood: the social construction of pregnancy and birth. In Kitzinger S, Davis J A (eds) The place of birth. Oxford University Press, Oxford

Richman J 1982 Men's experiences of pregnancy and childbirth. In McKee L, O'Brien M (eds) The father figure. Tavistock, London

Riviere P G 1974 The couvade: a problem reborn. Man   9: 424

Romalis C 1981 Taking care of the Little Woman: father-physician relations during pregnancy and childbirth. In Romalis S (ed) Childbirth – alternatives to medical control. University of Texas Press, Austin

Romito P 1986 The humanizing of childbirth: the response of medical institutions to women's demand for change. Midwifery   2: 135–40

Roopnarine J L, Miller B C 1985 Transitions to fatherhood. In Hanson S M H, Bozett F W (eds) Dimensions of fatherhood. Sage, Beverly Hills

Rothman B K 1982 In labour. Women and power in the birthplace. Norton, New York

Strickland O L 1987 The occurrence of symptoms in expectant fathers. Nursing Research   36 (3): 184–9

Thompson H 1982 What about father? Nursing Times, Community Outlook (April): 99–104

Trethowan W H, Conlon M F 1965 The couvade symptom. British Journal of Psychiatry   111: 57–66

Tylor E B 1865 Researches into the early history of mankind and the development of civilization, 2nd edn. John Murray, London

■ Suggested further reading

Chapman L 1991 Searching: expectant fathers' experiences during labor and birth. Journal of Perinatal and Neonatal Nursing   4 (4): 21–9

Jackson B 1984 Fatherhood. Allen and Unwin, London
Lamb M E 1986 The father's role: applied perspectives. John Wiley, New York
Lewis C 1986 Becoming a father. Open University Press, Milton Keynes
Russell G 1983 The changing role of fathers. Open University Press, Milton
    Keynes

Chapter 7

Safer motherhood – a midwifery challenge

Mary Kensington

> A Maternal Death is defined by the World Health Organisation (WHO) as the death of a woman while pregnant or within 42 days of termination of pregnancy, irrespective of the duration and the site of the pregnancy, from any cause related to or aggravated by the pregnancy or its management but not from accidental or incidental causes (WHO 1979).

The right of women to control their own fertility, receive care in pregnancy and enjoy successful childbirth is still denied to millions of women. This is reflected in the numbers of women who die in childbirth or who are severely injured in the process. In the developing world childbirth remains one of the leading causes of death in females between the ages of 14–45 (WHO 1987). The WHO estimates that there are 500 000 maternal deaths world wide each year of which 99 per cent occur in the developing world (WHO 1991). This tragedy is not only confined to the health of women and mothers but immediately affects the survival and quality of life of babies and children. There is also a long term effect on the woman's family and community with the loss of her economic productivity, and possibly even the disintegration of her family. Until recently this tragedy was largely ignored by the people who determined national and international health policies and it was the United Nations Decade for Women (1976–85) that put the focus on women's issues. This decade changed the emphasis on the issues of equality and human rights so that the topic of woman's health was finally recognised as a central development issue. There was an awakening to the fact that Health For All by the year 2000 (WHO 1978) was meaningless in the face of such losses due to maternal deaths, and the devastating fact that most of this death and suffering could have been avoided.

Since 1990, May 5th has been designated an annual International Day of the Midwife, but how aware are midwives in developed countries of the situation with regard to women and childbirth in developing countries?

The aim of this chapter is to provide the background information about the issues of maternal mortality and morbidity in developing countries that culminated in the Safe Motherhood Initiative. It is also to help the reader appreciate how the concept of safe motherhood challenges midwifery practice at international, national and community levels.

■ It is assumed you are already aware of the following:

- The definitions of *direct, indirect* and *fortuitous* maternal deaths (WHO 1979);

- The definition of maternal mortality rate;

- The definition of maternal morbidity;

- The 1985–1987 Report of Confidential Enquiries into Maternal Deaths in the United Kingdom (DoH 1991), or an equivalent enquiry in your own country.

- The history of maternity care in the United Kingdom (UK) or your own country and the reasons why maternal mortality in developed countries has been reduced dramatically within a short space of time.

■ The magnitude of the problem

□ Maternal mortality

Exact numbers of women who die as a result of pregnancy and childbirth each year are not known. Most of these women are poor and live in remote areas and often their deaths are not recorded. Many of these deaths take place outside hospital but, even where registration systems are established, problems have arisen through the incomplete or inaccurate recording of data. Often there is no mention of the cause of death (Royston & Armstrong 1989).

Most of the regional and worldwide statistics used to describe maternal deaths were formulated prior to the Safe Motherhood Conference in 1987 (WHO 1987; Zahr & Royston 1991). Since then there has been a great deal of new information resulting from detailed surveys at community level (WHO 1991).

When the percentage of live births worldwide by region are compared with the percentage of maternal deaths worldwide by region (see Fig. 7.2) an initial impression is gained of areas having the greatest potential for improvement. South Asia has 26.9 per cent and Africa 19.6 per cent of the

Figure 7.1 Case history supplied by Sister Anne Thompson, from her experience of working in The Cameroon

Mara was moribund when she was lifted down from the lorry which brought her to the district hospital. Her village was many miles away and the men had carried her in a hammock made from a blanket and slung on a pole, right through the forest and across the river until they found a lorry at the crossroads. She was lean and would have been elegant once, but now her skin was dry and rough, hot to the touch and putty coloured. Her mouth was dry and sore and her eyes rolled in unconsciousness. A greeny-black discharge poured from her vagina and it was hard not to recoil from the foul smell. The journey had been long, but they hadn't even started on the road until last night, three days after Mara had given birth to twins, with great difficulty and with no one trained to help.

In Mara's village, twins are not welcome – perhaps too often the problems which accompany their birth are interpreted as the power of evil spirits which come to harm the mother. Whatever the reason, tradition maintained that the old women, straight after the birth, counteract the work of the spirits by packing the birth canal with a paste made from an assortment of herbs, plants and, probably, less savoury substances. We had the story, bit by bit, over the next two days as we watched Mara die, from a young woman who had stayed with her. She did die, of course, despite our best efforts, our drips and antibiotics. And her death would only drive deeper the conviction of the older women that the birth of twins spells disaster.

world's live births but a massive 42.6 per cent and 38.4 per cent respectively of the maternal deaths. In comparison, Latin America's 9 per cent of the live births and 3.9 per cent of the maternal deaths appears favourable (Acsadi & Johnson-Acsadi 1990). By comparing the statistics of maternal deaths per 100 000 live births, however, the picture is made more clear. This is because people usually find it easier to visualise specific numbers rather than percentages. The figures also express the risk of death among women once they are pregnant. They can also be used for the planning of maternal and childbirth services (Royston & Armstrong 1989; Maine 1990). Figures 7.3 and 7.4 show the contrasts between 1983 and 1988 for maternal deaths per 100 000 live births. This latest information shows that pregnancy and childbirth has in fact become slightly safer for women in most of Asia and parts of Latin America. In contrast in most parts of sub-Saharan Africa the situation has not changed greatly for women where an increase in the number of births has led to a parallel increase in the number of maternal deaths. However results need to be interpreted with caution as it is not known which of the changes are real and which are due to better informa-

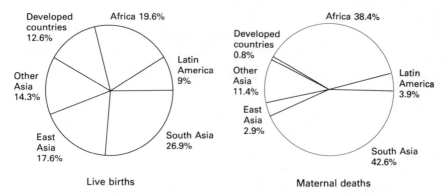

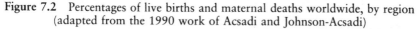

Figure 7.2 Percentages of live births and maternal deaths worldwide, by region (adapted from the 1990 work of Acsadi and Johnson-Acsadi)

tion systems (WHO 1991). Worldwide the number of maternal deaths has not changed greatly since 1983 (WHO 1991).

When maternal deaths in developing countries are compared with those in developed countries (Fig. 7.3) it is readily seen just how gross the disparities are. It is only by understanding a woman's lifetime risk of dying in pregnancy or childbirth, however, that one can begin to realise the magnitude of the problem at a more individual level. A woman's risk of dying is measured by

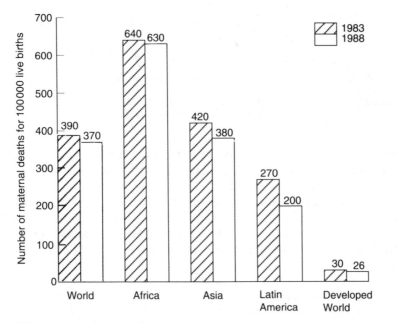

Figure 7.3 Estimated maternal deaths per 100 000 live births (adapted from WHO 1991)

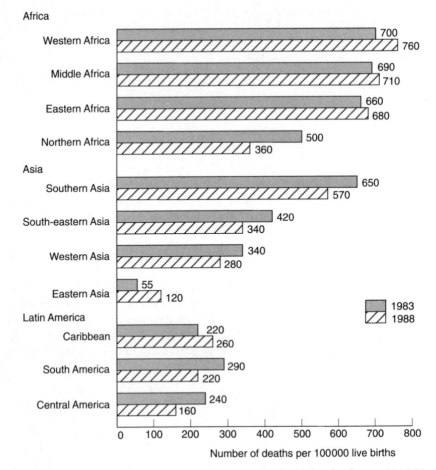

Figure 7.4. Estimated maternal mortality, 1983 and 1988 – deaths per 100 000 live births (adapted from WHO 1991)

the ratio of maternal deaths to live births as a result of a given pregnancy but her lifetime risk of maternal death will further depend on the numbers of times she becomes pregnant. For example for a woman in Southern Asia the average lifetime risk is 1 in 38 but for a woman in Africa it is 1 in 25 and in areas where fertility is high that risk may be as high as 1 in 15. For women in developed countries that risk is much lower – calculated as between 1:1 750 and 1:10 000 (Safe Motherhood 1989; Zahr & Royston 1991).

☐ **Maternal morbidity**

Data on morbidity is almost non-existent. However it is thought that for every woman who dies, about 16 other women suffer damage to their health which may last the rest of their lives (Royston & Armstrong 1989). Many of the problems women suffer as a result of childbirth under difficult conditions are related to obstructed labour, obstetric haemorrhage and puerperal sepsis (Royston & Armstrong 1989). The development of a fistula between the vagina and urethra or rectum, uterine prolapse and infertility are a few of the potential long term problems. Some of these women are so mutilated by childbirth that they are made social outcasts or even wish they had died (WHO 1987).

■ Causes of maternal deaths

Maternal mortality is said to be 'an indicator of [the level of] social inequity and discrimination against women' (WHO 1990:2), therefore it cannot be looked at only in terms of obstetric causes. A maternal death may be the end of a process that has influenced a woman's life since birth. Dr Fathalla portrayed the situation clearly when he used the metaphor of the Maternity Death Road (illustrated in Fig. 7.5) when addressing the Safe Motherhood Conference in Nairobi 1987 (WHO 1987).

In many countries behind the obstetric causes lies an inadequate health care system offering little or no antenatal care, due to lack of both trained personnel and essential supplies. Frequently there is delayed or no access to essential health care. In addition, there are the social, cultural, educational and political issues which determine the status of women, their health and fertility and whether they will seek health care. Surrounding the whole picture and influencing the outcome are the economic resources and infrastructure of the country.

□ Obstetric causes

It is usual to divide maternal deaths into three categories: direct, indirect and unrelated or fortuitous deaths (WHO 1979; DoH 1991). In developing countries the five major direct obstetric causes are haemorrhage (predominantly postpartum), sepsis, hypertension of pregnancy, obstructed labour and unsafe abortion (Kwast 1991). Indirect causes of maternal death are often due to concurrent illnesses including anaemia, malaria, viral hepatitis, rheumatic heart disease and the haemoglobinopathies (Zahr & Royston 1991).

The direct causes account for 75 per cent of maternal deaths and when anaemia is included this figure rises to 80 per cent (Maine 1990; Kwast 1991; Zahr & Royston 1991).

An important factor to be considered when looking at these figures is that all five of the major causes of maternal death have been drastically reduced with preventative and curative treatment in developed countries.

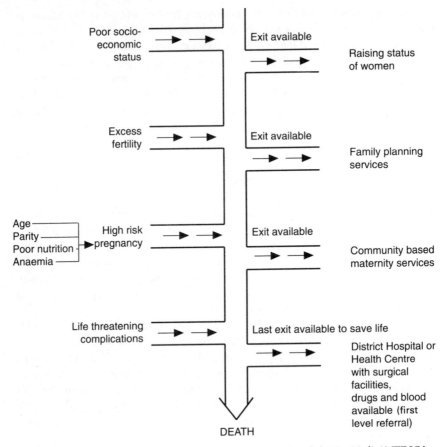

Figure 7.5 Maternity death road (adapted from 'Why did Mrs X die?' WHO's video explaining the concept of 'The Road to Maternal Death'. WHO 1989)

Another major contributory factor is that antenatal care is only available to a few. Over 50 per cent of the women do not have the assistance of any trained person in childbirth. In Southern Asia 25 per cent of women have trained help at delivery; Africa 38 per cent; Latin America 86 per cent; Eastern Asia 94 per cent and developed countries 99 per cent (Safe Motherhood 1989; Zahr & Royston 1991).

☐ **Reproductive factors**

Age and pregnancy order
It is well known that certain groups of women are more at risk during pregnancy and childbirth – girls of 15 years and under (Harrison 1985;

James 1989), women over 35 years (DoH 1991; Grant 1991), and those who have borne four or more children (DoH 1991; Grant 1991)

Women in Jamaica having their fifth to ninth birth were 43 per cent more likely to die than women having their second child and, in comparison with women aged 20–24 years, the risk of death was doubled for those in the 30–35 years age bracket and increased fivefold for women over 40 years (Walker *et al* 1986).

Girls under 15 years of age are five to seven times more likely to die in pregnancy and childbirth than women in the lowest risk group 20–24 years (Harrison 1985). In Niger 80 per cent of women with obstetric fistula resulting in urinary or faecal incontinence are between 15–19 years (Safe Motherhood 1989).

Harrison (1985) found that in the very young girl (15 years and under) there was a high incidence of eclampsia and obstructed labour whereas for the women of high parity (five or more previous children) obstetric haemorrhage caused greater maternal morbidity or death. Anaemia was a frequent finding and contributory factor in both groups. As might be expected Harrison (1985) also found that these high risk situations were usually related to conditions of poverty, poor environmental influences and a lack of or poor use of health facilities.

Birth spacing
This has been shown to have a strong relationship to the survival of children (Grant 1991) but there is conflicting evidence concerning whether closely spaced births (less than two years) have a measurable effect on the survival of the mother. Maine (1990) finds no evidence as yet to suggest this, but Grant (1991) sees births being too close as having a direct effect on maternal mortality figures.

Unwanted pregnancies
Women's improved access to family planning services, reducing the number of unwanted pregnancies and unsafe abortions, could be expected to have a major impact on reducing maternal mortality. Following analysis of the World Fertility Survey (carried out in the late 1970s) it was estimated 'that maternal deaths in many developing countries would be reduced by 25–40 per cent if all women who explicitly say that they want no more children were using a contraceptive method effectively' (WHO 1987: 35). The reality is that most women have no access to family planning services (WHO 1987; Royston & Armstrong 1989).

□ **Health behaviour and access to health services**

Access to health services is not a simple concept. Studies in developing countries reinforce the belief that a majority of maternal deaths could have

Figure 7.6   Case history supplied by Sister Anne Thompson, from her experience of working in The Cameroon

When Aissatou died giving birth to her fifth baby, the men of the village asked the midwife to come and explain to the family what had happened, for a number of them were determined to lynch her husband who was believed to have brought about her death. In fact, Aissatou, who lived fairly near the health centre, had set out on foot as soon as she realised she was bleeding, even though the pains had not started. She arrived at the centre alone, and a diagnosis of placenta praevia was made almost immediately. Arrangements were made to transport her in the Mayor's jeep to the district hospital so that a caesarean section could be performed. A lorry filled with relatives who had been coaxed and persuaded into giving blood trailed down the 60 miles of dirt road behind the jeep. Aissatou remained in good spirits through the journey despite her weakness (a dextrose/saline infusion is a poor substitute for blood if your haemoglobin is only about 7.5 g/dl to start with). Her baby's heartbeat remained steady, but so too did her blood loss. Confusion reigned at the hospital. The surgeon was absent on unexpected business. No one else was trained to perform even straightforward surgery. The family, 'captive' blood donors but most reluctant, quietly disappeared. It took Aissatou just four hours to die, undelivered, in her midwife's arms . . . not because of any spell which her poor husband was alleged to have cast upon her but because of a common, tragic combination of lack of resources, ignorance and fear.

been avoided with better access to services and with an improved standard of care and technology (Kwast 1990; Maine 1990).

Bullough (1981) and Harrison (1985) show in their studies that many women who died in health centres or hospitals had arrived in very poor condition and that most had never received any antenatal care. 'Delay' has emerged as a strong contributing factor to maternal deaths. Thaddeus and Maine (1990) in their book *Too Far To Walk* have developed a conceptual framework to look at three phases of delay as a way of highlighting the factors involved.

Phase 1   This considers factors that affect a woman's decision to seek care. These include her status within the family, whether she has decision making power, her financial situation and her perception of her own health or illness.

Phase 2   This looks at factors that contribute to delay in arriving at a health care facility. These include access to transport, previous experience of the health centre and distribution of health facilities.

Phase 3   This deals with delay in receiving adequate care at the health care facility.

☐ Socioeconomic factors

One of the most important factors affecting Safe Motherhood is the low status of women. Where socioeconomic conditions are poor and the environmental conditions harsh (rural areas, urban slums), women and girls are disadvantaged and discriminated against through neglect, repression and ignorance (Jeffery *et al* 1989; Momsen 1991).

- They have less food than boys and men and this leads to malnutrition, anaemia and ill health;

- They receive less care than boys and men during sickness;

- Girls have less chance than boys of going to school;

- Women work longer hours than their menfolk and carry a double burden of work at home and in the fields;

- Women lack employment opportunity and therefore income;

- Girls are often forced to marry young and in some cultures the father/husband has complete authority over the woman so that even if she becomes ill no one else will make the decision to get help if the man is away (Mahler 1987; Safe Motherhood July 1989; Grant 1991).

The interrelationship between socioeconomic factors and pregnancy and childbirth has already been highlighted under the section on reproductive factors, but what effect does education have?

Reviews of studies by Thaddeus and Maine (1990) show that the role of education is not clear but it does appear that with increasing levels of education the medical services were utilised more. Other reports showed a direct correlation between improved education of women and the health of all family members including a greater uptake of family planning services. Most importantly women's earning capacity and therefore their power in decision making increased giving them equal opportunity and higher status (Harrison 1985; Rosenfeld 1989; Safe Motherhood July 1991).

The factors predisposing to maternal deaths are complex and interrelated. It is impossible to isolate the single most significant factor but, by focusing on a few, maternal mortality figures can be reduced dramatically. Sri Lanka is one place where this has been achieved. Over the last 40 years as a result of a programme concentrating on the education of women, provision of family planning services and trained assistance at births, Sri Lanka succeeded in reducing maternal mortality from 580 per 100 000 live

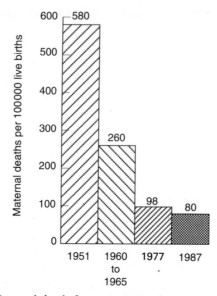

Figure 7.7 Maternal death figures in Sri Lanka per 100 000 live births

births in 1951 to 80 in 1987 (see Fig. 7.7) (Royston & Armstrong 1989; Zahr & Royston 1991).

■ The Safe Motherhood Initiative

The United Nations Decade for Women (1976–85) made people aware that women's health issues had received too little attention and there was a need to consider women separately from men when planning for development.

An important outcome of this decade was the Safe Motherhood Initiative (SMI) which was developed during the Safe Motherhood Conference held in Nairobi, Kenya in February 1987. This international conference, co-sponsored by WHO, the World Bank and the United Nations Fund for Population Activities (UNFPA), was the first to focus specifically on women. The unanimous agreement was a global commitment to reduce by 50 per cent the rate of maternal mortality by the year 2000.

The major objectives of the Initiative are:

1. Raising women's socioeconomic, legal and educational status.

2. Increasing women's access to family planning services.

3. Improving routine care during pregnancy, childbirth and the postpartum period. This includes the assistance of trained personnel for all women in childbirth whether at home or in hospital.

4. Improving the accessibility and quality of treatment for obstetric
   emergencies.

   (WHO 1987)

Each objective alone would improve the quality of life and health of girls
and women, however the goal of Safer Motherhood can only be achieved if
a broad strategy is used combining each of the four major objectives.

■ The midwifery challenge

The Safe Motherhood Conference report (WHO 1987) rarely mentions the
midwife or what her role could be. The report focuses mainly on the
community health worker (CHW) and traditional birth attendant (TBA)
and the structures needed for changes in health and society in order to
reduce maternal mortality and morbidity.

However, the issue of Safe Motherhood is at the core of midwifery
practice. A midwife has chosen to be with a woman at one of the most
crucial events of her life.

> She accept[s] through education/training the responsibility of caring
> for women throughout their reproductive years and to concern
> herself with promotive and preventative health action in families and
> in communities. Safe Motherhood is therefore her only concern.
>
> (WHO/ICM 1987:2)

In order to achieve the main objectives of the SMI, midwives have had to
ask themselves questions. What is the midwives' role and function? Is their
education appropriate to meet the goals of Safe Motherhood? Are there
enough midwives? To what extent can midwives change the situation?
(Kwast 1990).

The section which follows looks at the midwifery response at an international,
national and community level.

□ International action

The International Confederation of Midwives (ICM) was the first inter-
national organisation to take up the challenge of the Safe Motherhood
Conference. Six months after the Nairobi Conference, in August 1987, the
ICM held a workshop in conjunction with WHO and United Nations
Children's Fund (UNICEF) on 'Women's Health and the Midwife: A Global
Perspective' in The Hague, Netherlands. The result of this was the formulation

of specific midwifery actions to promote maternal health and reduce maternal mortality and morbidity – that is to make Safe Motherhood Initiatives.

The challenge was to push forward initiatives that were already in existence and to create new ones particularly in developing countries (WHO/ICM 1987). The outcome of this workshop was a statement from midwives all over the world that they were committed to collective action.

As a way of analysing the problems and developing a strategy for action four areas were looked at. There was a recognition that change was needed in relation to the following.

1. Education, both basic and post basic, with an emphasis on problem solving and a community based training
It was realised that there was a shortage of midwives and that, while most worked in hospitals in large towns, the highest number of maternal deaths occurred in the rural areas or urban slum dwellings. It was appreciated that the city midwife would not be familiar with rural women and their problems and often was not willing to work in the countryside (Bentley 1987; Kwast 1990). It appeared vital to develop a training programme that would prepare midwives to be more community based and able to support and supervise other community based providers of maternity care. It also appeared important to help people in the community to develop strategies to maintain their own health.

2. Extending the role and function of midwives
If the major causes of maternal death were to be confronted midwives needed training and authority to perform obstetric life saving procedures. For example administration of intravenous fluids, manual removal of the placenta, and administration of drugs to treat severe pre-eclampsia and eclampsia (WHO/ICM1987).

3. Administration and management
The importance of reallocating staff and restructuring services was realised especially in the face of the serious shortage of midwives. The need to identify and appraise resources was also highlighted (WHO/ICM 1987).

4. Midwifery research
There was increased awareness that midwives at all levels need to collect, analyse and interpret data so that the resources can be centred in areas of greatest need (WHO/ICM 1987).

Since the workshop in The Hague 1987, the ICM has held others to help prepare midwives for their new role, and to explore and plan through a structured process what action will be needed to help reduce maternal mortality and morbidity within their own nation (ICM/WHO 1989).

The first was held in January 1989 in Ghana entitled 'Enhancing National

Midwifery Services'. Teams from Ghana, the Gambia, Liberia, Nigeria and Sierra Leone were involved. They were asked to produce a plan for introducing changes within the constraints of their existing health services and the situation within their country. The specific actions outlined were to be undertaken by midwives but the issues considered were to relate to all maternity care providers – for example (ICM/WHO 1989):

- To introduce to clients, TBAs and to the community the concept of 'At Risk' coding for pregnant women;

- To introduce use of the partograph to reduce the large number of prolonged labours (with the sequelae of vesico-vaginal or recto-vaginal fistula, sepsis and mortality).

Two other workshops run by the ICM and also held in 1989 were a two day workshop in Hong Kong ('The Midwife – The Key to Safe Motherhood') and later in the year in Germany a workshop on midwifery and research. A similar workshop to the one held in Ghana was held in January 1990 and was the first Francophone workshop. It took place in Burkino Faso with eight West African countries being invited (WHO/ICM 1991).

The next major workshop was held in October 1990 in Kobe, Japan. Entitled 'Midwifery Education: Action for Safe Motherhood' it was run by the ICM, WHO and UNICEF. This workshop was not only to evaluate the progress with regards to maternal mortality and morbidity since 1987 but also to develop new strategies for coping with this problem. The Kobe workshop marked a turning point for the ICM. The reality is that maternal mortality figures remain virtually unchanged and midwifery is in a crisis situation with insufficient midwives to support the community level and to provide essential life saving skills (WHO/ICM 1991). It was recognised that the goal of reducing maternal mortality by 50 per cent could not be achieved in nine years unless a more decisive strategy was developed and instigated at grass roots level, in addition to continuing to effect changes at the highest levels within countries and national organisations.

Education is a key area to target if long term changes are to be made to reduce maternal mortality and morbidity. Education can become the 'practice of freedom' as Freire (1972) an educationalist in Brazil found. His methods challenged the people (mostly peasants) to question their lives and to find ways to solve their own problems and transform their society. Midwives (and communities) need to develop a similar strategy to deal with the realities of their day to day lives.

The Kobe workshop also reflected the growth (since 1987) of confidence among midwives who had moved from *thinking* that they might have the ability and skill to deal effectively with maternal health problems to now *believing* that they do. This increase in confidence is reflected in the language used. In 1987 it was satted that 'the midwife *could be* the key' to reducing maternal mortality and morbidity (Bentley 1987). At Kobe the words were 'the midwife is the key, the linchpin' (Kwast & Bentley 1991). This awakening process and growth of confidence was vital in their production of a plan that would allow the introduction of competent and confident midwives who would be central to the success of the maternity care team and thus realise their own potential. The midwife would be trained to be the team leader for those involved in the community maternity care and would be the link between the community and the district level hospital (WHO/ ICM 1991). To achieve this, the Kobe workshop outlined the necessary educational changes and stressed the following points.

1. The importance of using a problem solving approach

There was a recognition that there is a shortage of midwife teachers; that teaching styles were outdated and resources inadequate. Methodology of teaching adopted from developed countries is often not appropriate in other areas (WHO/ICM 1991). Midwives' training should reflect realistic needs of the local community and prepare midwives to cope with problems as they arise, as specialist referral is not readily accessible.

2. The need to get rid of the nursing model, which is based on ill health, and to put an emphasis on promotive and preventative health (WHO/ICM 1991)

There was a recognition that many developing countries have integrated midwifery and nursing training in the hope of producing a more generalist nurse who is able to work in all areas and therefore is more cost effective. However if maternal mortality is to be truly challenged then specialist midwives are needed (Kwast 1990).

3. The importance of a community based training

This was seen not only as a way to attract midwives to rural areas (where there is an acute shortage) and thereby increase primary health services but also to close the gap between community maternity care (mostly provided by TBAs) and the first referral level midwives at the district hospital (WHO/ ICM 1991).

The emphasis of the workshop was to provide a forum for discussion about ways of directly affecting a reduction in the major causes of maternal mortality. The ongoing effect would also be to influence maternal morbidity figures and to reduce perinatal mortality and childhood morbidity. Hence the outcome of the Kobe workshop was the production of a basic educational framework which could be used immediately for curriculum development and was related to the five major causes of maternal mortality. Each cause was addressed under the headings of community, prevention, treatment and follow up as a way of ensuring that midwives understood what was necessary to be able to deal more effectively with each major cause (WHO/ICM 1991).

Action began soon after the workshop when Gaynor Maclean (a midwifery educator in Wales who was a facilitator at the workshop in Kobe) was appointed by the WHO specifically to prepare learning packages using a modular approach. The construction of these learning packages is an exciting development in midwifery and provides a chance for midwives to be at the forefront of organising maternity care teams and having an impact on maternal mortality in rural areas. For the midwifery educators there is the opportunity to make safe practice a real possibility, as well as interesting and stimulating learning. The packages are devised with booklets, fact sheets, visual aids, exercises, games, articles and references (Maclean 1992). In order to increase the confidence and competence of midwives Maclean (1991) emphasises throughout the learning packages the importance of making links between theory and practice, cause and effect, process and outcome, and also stresses the difference that appropriate intervention can make.

This use of the problem solving approach will ensure midwives become increasingly critical of the situation in which they themselves live, and are challenged to find answers. The exciting consequence of this, one would hope, is that midwives will act as change agents in encouraging people in the community to instigate changes to improve their own health and standard of living.

Gaynor Maclean has begun the pre-testing of these learning packages at pilot centres in Botswana in September 1991 and results are proving to be very encouraging (Maclean & Tickner 1992).

☐ **National action**

Tanzania – where maternal mortality is estimated at 340 per 100 000 live births (Grant 1991) – was the first country to take action following the workshop in Kobe. Stella Mpanda, a midwife who participated at the workshop, returned to her country enthused and set about organising a National workshop. She gathered together midwives from clinical areas and education, influential people in nursing and medicine, and representatives from the government. The workshop was held in September 1991 and addressed midwifery education and practice issues directed towards implementing Safe Motherhood Initiatives in Tanzania. The outcome of the workshop was the understanding that the midwife has the primary responsibility for developing and supervising maternity care, together with the acceptance that midwifery education must be community based, and that the goal of reducing maternal mortality and morbidity can only be realised by improving care and participation at the community level (Tickner 1991).

To achieve this goal a number of recommendations were made that show the commitment of Tanzanian midwives and government officials to achieving Safer Motherhood by ensuring the midwife's position is strengthened through the development of midwifery education, practice and research. This was an important development in a country where there did not appear to be existing legislation or policies to support midwives in their practice (Tickner 1991).

It is to be hoped that such commitment will inspire midwives in other countries to take such action.

☐ **Community action**

One innovative and exciting example of midwifery action at a local community level is the Magbil project. Magbil is a large village in the Port Loko District in Sierra Leone and is surrounded by many smaller villages.

In Sierra Leone, 68 per cent of the population live in rural areas and maternal mortality is estimated at 450 per 100 000 live births (Grant 1991). Poverty is an everyday reality for these women in the rural areas, where there are inadequate freshwater supplies, poor roads with little or no transport, high rates of illiteracy and a lack of medical facilities (Grant 1991).

In 1989, Isha Daramy-Kabia (a midwife) realised a vision she had had of setting up a community health centre in the village of Magbil – to improve the health and lives of women and their families, and to train TBAs. Magbil was established as a pilot project and with community support the health centre was opened in June 1990. An additional piece of land was also provided and the women were given education in market gardening and the growing of cash crops so that ultimately the centre could become self-financing (Daramy-Kabia 1989).

The first part of this dream became a reality. The project was then expanded to fulfil the second aim of improving maternal and child health in Magbil and the surrounding villages by midwives training and working alongside TBAs (Daramy-Kabia 1992).

In Sierra Leone over 60 per cent of deliveries are carried out by TBAs whether trained or not (Daramy-Kabia 1989). As discussed earlier this is a common feature of developing countries.

Until recently there has been a great deal of emphasis on the training of TBAs as it was thought that this was the answer to reducing maternal deaths, but there has been little or no change in maternal mortality rates. This has resulted in much argument concerning the continuation of TBA training (Leedham 1985; Bullough 1989; Harrison 1989, 1990). The reality, however, is that the majority of deliveries are conducted by TBAs and will continue to be so for years to come. Until a qualified midwife is available for each delivery then the TBA is needed and cannot be ignored.

In the past the TBA training has been limited as there have been no midwives either to support them, nor at the first referral level for TBAs to refer to (Kwast 1991; Safe Motherhood 1991). With the emphasis on midwifery training becoming community based this situation will be slowly rectified.

Projects like that at Magbil are very important because they recognise firstly that the TBA is a vital link between the midwife and the community (for she knows the community and its beliefs and is accepted by the women) and secondly that the midwife must be the person who trains, supports and supervises the TBA. Twenty-two TBAs covering eighteen villages, have now completed an eight month training programme with Isha Daramy-Kabia, and been awarded certificates and delivery kits (Daramy-Kabia 1992). The next project is the provision of birthing rooms in each village where the TBAs work, in order that they may keep up the high standard of care they learned in Magbil (Brain 1992).

The progression and development of a critical awareness within the midwifery profession internationally, nationally and locally is inspiring and forward looking. Many other examples exist to show that action is being taken worldwide to achieve safer motherhood through establishing and strengthening the maternity care team and with the introduction of tools such as the partograph, home based maternal records and the use of maternity waiting homes – low-cost shelters close to the district hospital where pregnant women considered to be high risk can stay prior to the onset of labour (WHO 1987).

■ Conclusions

This chapter is not just about the situation in developing countries; developed and developing countries are not separate worlds with their own unique sets of problems. The principles discussed here apply also to developed countries. Maternal mortality figures may be low there but there are still disparities between regions (DoH 1991), and between ethnic groups (DoH 1989). Improvements are still needed. Maternal morbidity remains very much an unknown, undocumented subject within developed countries, and this is a problem which needs to be addressed (WHO 1985).

Current developments in the United Kingdom include the problem solving approach to education and transferring the emphasis of midwifery training and practice into the community. Even in developed countries, the overall aim should be to increase the numbers of competent and confident midwives who respond to their communities, have knowledge of epidemiology and research, who have teaching and management skills and are able to act as advocates for their clients.

The midwifery challenge continues worldwide to work towards Safer Motherhood.

■ **Recommendations for clinical practice in the light of currently available evidence**

1. Midwives should ensure that they are aware of the major causes of maternal death in the country in which they are practising, and should consider what they themselves can do to reduce maternal mortality and morbidity.

2. In the light of the recommendations of successive Reports on Confidential Enquiries into Maternal Deaths in England and Wales, midwives should ensure that all general anaesthetics in their unit are performed by a senior registrar or consultant anaesthetist.

3. All maternity units should have a protocol for management of fulminating pre-eclampsia and have access to a regional specialist unit (DoH 1991).

4. Midwives need to be up to date concerning what is happening to the family planning services in their area and in the United Kingdom. They should be aware that proposed changes may affect services and standards of care for women, especially those from disadvantaged areas and cultural minority backgrounds.

5. Midwives should be aware of what the law and practice is regarding female circumcision in the United Kingdom or their own country. (For the UK, refer to the Prohibition of Female Circumcision Act 1985, and also to the Foundation for Women's Health, Research and Development, who are carrying out an enquiry into the extent and practice of female genital mutilation.)

6. The goal of safer motherhood extends to all. Midwives should know about the 'Safer childbirth for travellers' campaign (see the Useful addresses list at the end of this chapter) and understand why there is a need to offer such a service in the United Kingdom.

7. Currently, the aim of midwifery training and practice in the United Kingdom is to give as much care in the community as possible (HC 1992). Midwives need to be involved in ensuring that this process continues to happen, and to look closely at how it is working.

8. Midwives need to foster links with other health groups to look at further strategies which could be developed to increase awareness on the part of both women and men that the achievement of health requires a change in individual health behaviours as well as an understanding of the social and environmental changes required. This will improve the health both of women and of children.

9. Midwives should be debating and discussing whether developing countries should be looking to the West for answers. This is

particularly relevant given the increased use of technology in maternity care in the developed world.

■ Practice check

- Look at maternal deaths in the United Kingdom by region (DoH 1991) and ethnic group (DoH 1989). What explanation would you suggest for the differences which exist? What further research do you think should be carried out?

- It is important constantly to question your own practice and that in your unit. Is it safe? Is it research-based? For example, can you always justify your decision to perform an artificial rupture of the membranes (Henderson 1990)? Does your unit policy allow women in labour to eat and drink (Grant 1990)? Are you aware of the debate concerning the use of forceps versus ventouse (Vacca 1992)?

- Does your unit use a partograph? Do you think it is an important midwifery tool?

- How do you manage the third stage of normal labour? Should midwives continue to encourage physiological management or instigate further research into the debate of active versus physiological management in the third stage of normal labour (Levy 1990)?

- Are you confident in your knowledge and practice with regard to resuscitation of pregnant women? Is regular instruction given in your unit?

□ Acknowledgements

I would like to thank Gaynor Maclean midwifery consultant for the WHO SMI, Anne Thompson lecturer at the Royal College of Midwives and Jo Alexander series editor for this book, for their advice, suggestions and encouragement. I am also indebted to my midwifery colleagues Kate Lush and Jenny Fleming for their support and help in improving the structure of the text. Thanks are also due to Isha Daramy-Kabia for her kind permission to use her project proposal, and to the World Health Organisation for permission to reproduce Fig. 7.4, taken from WHO Weekly Epidemiology Rec. No. 47 1991, and to use information from Valerie Tickner's report on Safe Motherhood in Tanzania.

■ References

Acsadi G T, Johnson-Acsadi G 1990 Safe Motherhood in South Asia: socio-cultural and demographic aspects of maternal health. Background paper for Safe Motherhood South Asia Conference, Lahore, Pakistan

Bentley J 1987 Maternal mortality and morbidity – a midwifery challenge. Paper presented at the pre-congress workshop: Women's health and the midwife: a global perspective. WHO/ICM, Geneva

Brain M 1992 A New Year's message from the Royal College of Midwives president. Midwives Chronicle 105 (1248): 2

Bullough C 1981 Analysis of maternal deaths in the central region of Malawi. Reprinted 1990. In Thaddeus S, Maine D (eds) Too far to walk. Center for Population and Community Health, New York

Bullough C 1989 Maternal mortality in developing countries. British Journal of Obstetrics and Gynaecology 96: 1119–20

Daramy-Kabia I 1989 Magbil project proposal. Unpublished

Daramy-Kabia I 1992 Personal communication with the author in January

Department of Health 1989 Report on confidential enquiries into maternal deaths in England and Wales 1982–1984. HMSO, London

Department of Health 1991 Report on confidential enquiries into maternal deaths in the United Kingdom 1985–1987. HMSO, London

Fathalla M 1989 Why did Mrs X die? WHO's video explaining the concept of 'The road to maternal death'. WHO, Geneva

Freire P 1972 Pedagogy of the oppressed. Penguin, London

Grant J 1990 Nutrition and hydration in labour. In Alexander J, Levy V, Roch S (eds) Intrapartum care: a research-based approach (Midwifery Practice, Vol 2). Macmillan, Basingstoke.

Grant J 1991 The state of the world's children. Published for UNICEF, Oxford University Press, Oxford

Harrison K 1985 Childbearing, health and social priorities. British Journal of Obstetrics and Gynaecology 92 (Supplement 5): 1–119

Harrison K 1989 Maternal mortality in developing countries. Commentary. British Journal of Obstetrics and Gynaecology 96: 1–3; 1121–3

Harrison K 1990 Author's reply. British Journal of Obstetrics and Gynaecology 97: 87–92

Henderson C 1990 Artificial rupture of the membranes. In Alexander J, Levy V, Roch S (eds) Intrapartum care: a research-based approach (Midwifery Practice, Vol 2). Macmillan, Basingstoke

House of Commons (HC) Health Committee 1992 Report on the maternity services (Winterton Report). HMSO, London

ICM/WHO 1989 Planning for action by midwives. Report of a workshop on 'Enhancing national midwifery services' held in Accra, Ghana. International Confederation of Midwives, London.

James D 1989 High risk pregnancies. In Studd J (ed) Progress in obstetrics and gynaecology, Vol 7. Churchill Livingstone, London and Edinburgh

Jeffery P, Jeffery R, Lyon A 1989 Labour pains and labour power: women and childbearing in India. Zed Books, London

Kwast B 1990 Midwifery and safe motherhood. In Fagin C (ed) Nursing leadership: global strategy. National League For Nursing, New York

Kwast B 1991 Maternal mortality: the magnitude and the causes. Midwifery 7 (1): 4–7

Kwast B, Bentley J 1991 Introducing confident midwives: midwifery education – action for safe motherhood. Midwifery 7 (1): 8–19

Leedham E 1985 Traditional birth attendants. International Journal of Gynaecology and Obstetrics 23: 249–74

Levy V 1990 The midwife's management of the third stage of labour. In Alexander J, Levy V, Roch S (eds) Intrapartum care: a research-based approach (Midwifery Practice, Vol 2). Macmillan, Basingstoke

Maclean G 1991 Personal communication with the author in April

Maclean G 1992 Daring to care for women at risk. A report of the WHO Safe Motherhood Initiative: educational project. Paper presented at the first RCM student midwives conference, November 1991. Midwives Chronicle 105 (1258): 354–8

Maclean G, Tickner V 1992 A preliminary evaluation of education material prepared for the Safe Motherhood Initiative Educational Project. Midwifery 8 (3): 143–8

Mahler H 1987 The Safe Motherhood Initiative: a call to action. Lancet 1: 668–70

Maine D 1990 Safe motherhood programs: options and issues. Center for Population and Family Health, New York

Momsen J H 1991 Women and development in the Third World. Routledge, London

Rosenfeld A 1989 Maternal mortality in developing countries. Journal of the American Medical Association 262 (3): 367–79

Royston E, Armstrong S (eds) 1989 Preventing maternal deaths. WHO, Geneva

Safe Motherhood 1989 Newsletter Issue 1: 6, 7 November. Division of Family Health. WHO, Geneva

Safe Motherhood 1991 Newsletter Issue 5:9 March; Issue 6:5, 6 July. Division of Family Health. WHO, Geneva

Thaddeus S, Maine D 1990 Too far to walk: maternal mortality in context. Center for Population and Family Health, Columbia University, New York

Tickner V 1991 Report of the workshop/seminar on midwifery education for safe motherhood in Iringa, Tanzania, March 4–8. RCM, London. Unpublished

Vacca A 1992 A handbook of vacuum extraction. Edward Arnold, Sevenoaks

Walker G, Ashley D, McCaw A, Bernard G 1986 Maternal mortality in Jamaica. Lancet 1: 486–8

WHO 1978 Alma-Ata 1978 Primary health care. WHO, Geneva

WHO 1979 International classification of diseases, injuries and causes of death (ICD–9). WHO, Geneva

WHO 1985 Having a baby in Europe. WHO, Copenhagen

WHO 1987 Preventing the tragedy of maternal deaths: report on the International Safe Motherhood Conference, Kenya. World Bank, WHO and United Nations Fund for Population Activities

WHO 1990 Maternal health and safe motherhood programme: a progress report. WHO Maternal Child Health, Geneva

WHO 1991 Weekly Epidemiology Records, No. 47: 345–8. WHO, Geneva

WHO/ICM 1987 Women's health and the midwife: a global perspective. Report of a collaborative pre-congress workshop, The Hague, Netherlands (August 21–22) WHO/Maternal Child Health, Geneva

WHO/ICM 1991 Midwifery education: action for safe motherhood. Report of a collaborative pre-congress workshop, Kobe, Japan (October 5–6) WHO/Maternal Child Health, Geneva

Zahr C, Royston E 1991 Maternal mortality: a global factbook. WHO, Geneva. Chapter 2: 3–15

■ Suggested further reading

Bullough C, Lennox C, Lawson J 1989 Maternity care in developing countries. Proceedings of obstetricians and gynaecologists (June–July 1989) RCOG, London

Kelly J 1991 Fistulae of obstetric origin. Midwifery 7 (2): 71–3

Kwast B 1991 Postpartum haemorrhage: its contribution to maternal mortality. Midwifery 7 (2): 64–70

Kwast B 1991 Puerperal sepsis: its contribution to maternal mortality. Midwifery 7 (3): 102–106

Kwast B 1991 The hypertensive disorders of pregnancy: their contribution to maternal mortality. Midwifery 7 (4): 155–61

Kwast B 1991 Safe Motherhood: a challenge to midwifery practice. Round Table World Health Forum 12 (1): 1–24. WHO, Geneva

Kwast B 1992 Obstructed labour: its contribution to maternal mortality. Midwifery 8 (1): 3–7

Kwast B 1992 Abortion: its contribution to maternal mortality. Midwifery 8 (1): 8–11

Loudon I 1986 Obstetric care, social class and maternal mortality. British Medical Journal 293: 606–608

Maclean G 1992 Helping midwives in developing countries. Nursing Standard 6 (32): 25–7

Peters M 1988 A challenge for midwives: the reduction of maternal mortality and morbidity rates throughout the world. Midwifery 4 (1): 3–8

Pietila H, Vickers J 1990 Making women matter: the role of the United Nations. Zed Books, London

Starrs A, Measham D 1990 Challenge for the nineties. Safe Motherhood in South Asia. Report of conference held in Lahore, Pakistan (March 24–28). The World Bank and Family Care International

■ Useful addresses

Centre for International Child Health
Institute of Child Health
30 Guildford Street
London WC1N 1EH

Courses held:
Certificate in Safer Motherhood and Perinatal Health (six week course for senior midwives and obstetric nurses working in developing countries)
MSc in Mother and Child Health (14 months course designed for health professionals who already have experience of working in developing countries)

Center for Population and Family Health
Columbia University
60 Haven Avenue B–3
New York
NY 10032

International Confederation of Midwives
10 Barley Mow Passage
Chiswick
London W4
081 994 6477

Foundation for Women's Health Research and Development (FORWARD)
38 King Street
London
WC2E 8JT

Safer Childbirth for Travellers
$^c/_o$ 3rd floor
Jadwin House
205–211 Kentish Town Road
London
NW5 2JU
071 267 6723/4

Safe Motherhood Newsletter (free subscription)
Issued by the Division of Family Health
World Health Organisation
1211 Geneva 27
Switzerland

Chapter 8

Pain and the neonate

Valerie Fletcher

Advances in medical and nursing practice over the past decade have greatly improved the prognosis for low birthweight and sick newborn infants. The day-to-day management of these infants, however, necessitates frequent investigations and interventions – be they invasive or non-invasive. Many procedures also disturb the infant's rest.

The assessment and treatment of infant pain is a major clinical problem, and represents a monumental challenge to neonatal nurses and midwives. Sick or low birthweight babies do not possess language and are often intubated or paralysed, thus their verbal and behavioural responses to painful stimuli may be inhibited (Frank 1989). In practice, there may be lack of knowledge and general disagreement amongst medical and nursing staff as to the appropriate clinical signs and physiological measures indicative of pain and discomfort in infants. In addition, pain assessment and management are made more difficult by the apparent physiological and psychological immaturity of the neonate and the busy, noisy environment of the neonatal intensive care unit.

Recent evidence suggests that infants do experience pain and may, indeed, be hypersensitive to painful procedures (Fitzgerald *et al* 1989). Many health professionals, however, choose to ignore infants' potential to feel pain or expect them to have an adult perspective. Personal bias, lack of sensitivity or empathy and inability to view a tiny baby as an individual with needs and rights, may contribute to inadequate management of infant pain (Fletcher 1990).

■ **It is assumed that you are already aware of the following:**

• The characteristics of the healthy, term baby;

• The characteristics of the preterm baby;

• The commonly held theories of pain and its perception (Wall & Melzack 1984)

134

■ Nociceptive activity and the neonate

> The focus on pain perception in neonates and confusion over its differentiation from nociceptive activity and the accompanying physiologic responses have obscured the mounting evidence that nociception is important in the biology of the neonate. This is true regardless of any philosophical view on consciousness and pain perception in newborns.
>
> (Anand & Hickey 1987)

The evaluation of pain in the human fetus and neonate is difficult because pain is generally defined as a subjective phenomenon. Our understanding of the mechanisms underlying pain has increased significantly in recent years (Wall & Melzack 1984). In the literature relating specifically to the neonate, terms relating to pain and nociception are used interchangeably, but in this chapter 'nociceptive activity' is preferred as the word 'pain' has strong emotive associations.

Nociceptors are receptors which respond to harmful stimuli. They are found in skin, muscle, viscera and other tissues. Any tissue damage results in the release of substances – for example histamine, bradykinin and potassium – which sensitise nociceptors to other stimuli. Prostaglandins are also released and potentiate the effects of these substances. Nociceptors convert this activity into electrical stimuli (a process known as 'transducing') which send 'pain messages' to the brain.

There are two types of nociceptors; each has different properties.

- *The high threshold mechanoceptor* responds rapidly at the site of stimulation. The receptor ending is simple and the afferent axon (leading to the spinal cord) is a thinly mylenated A delta fibre. These are responsible for the initial sharp sensation of pain registered as simultaneous with the injury.

- *The polymodal nociceptor* responds to various stimuli including noxious heat (above 43 °C), intense mechanical stimulation and irritant chemicals. The polymodal nociceptors, which are very common, are innervated by unmylenated C fibres. These conduct stimuli slowly resulting in a more prolonged and lasting sensation.

The belief that infants are incapable of experiencing pain is founded on the following assumptions: that incomplete mylenation of the peripheral nerves (A delta fibres) means that pain is not felt; that C fibres are few in neonates; and that the central nervous system of the infant is underdeveloped. The following discussion will address these issues.

☐ **Anatomical perspectives**

• *Assumption 1 – Preterm infants lack mylenation of the peripheral nerves meaning that immediate, sharp responses are not registered properly*
Lack of mylenation has been proposed as an index of the lack of maturity in the neonatal nervous system and is used to support the argument that preterm and full term infants are not capable of pain perception (Owens 1984). Incomplete mylenation implies a slower conduction velocity in the nerve tracts of neonates. Anand and Hickey (1987), however, suggest that this may be misleading as the comparative size of the neonatal nervous system more than compensates for any reduced speed of conduction. Furthermore, quantitative neuroanatomical data (Gleiss & Stuttgen 1970) have shown that nociceptive nerve tracts in the central nervous system undergo complete mylenation during the second and third trimester of gestation. This would suggest that assumptions about inability to feel pain made on the basis of lack of mylenation may not be reliable.

• *Assumption 2 – C fibres are few in neonates*
The neural pathways for pain may be traced from sensory receptors in the skin to sensory areas in the cerebral cortex of newborn infants. Contrary to widespread belief, the density of nociceptive nerve endings in the skin of newborns is similar to, or greater than, that in adult skin (Gleiss & Stuttgen 1970).

• *Assumption 3 – The central nervous system of the infant is underdeveloped leading to inadequate transmission of stimuli to the brain*
Functional maturity of the cerebral cortex is suggested by fetal and neonatal electroencephalographic patterns, studies of cerebral metabolism and the behavioural development of neonates. At 20 weeks gestation, activity can be seen in both cerebral hemispheres. These bursts of activity have been found to be sustained by 22 weeks gestation (Spehlmann 1981). By 30 weeks, the distinction between wakefulness and sleep can be made on the basis of EEG patterns (Spehlmann 1981). Cortical components of visually and auditorily evoked potentials have been recorded in preterm babies born before 30 weeks gestation (Henderson-Smart *et al* 1983; Torres & Anderson 1985).
Olfactory and tactile stimuli may also cause detectable changes in EEG patterns of neonates (Spehlmann 1981). In addition, several forms of behaviour imply cortical activity during intrauterine life. Well defined periods of quiet sleep, active sleep and wakefulness occur *in utero* beginning at 28 weeks gestation (Arduini *et al* 1986).

■ Infants' perception of pain: how does it differ from adults'?

□ Investigating responses to stimuli

One method of investigating the effect of sensory inputs is to look at the motor responses they evoke. These responses also reflect the activity in the motor neurones and muscle as well as in the sensory pathways, however, and may not necessarily reflect sensory experience (Fitzgerald *et al* 1988).

Cutaneous reflexes (an automatic and purposeful withdrawal of the limb or affected area away from the offending stimuli) have been used to establish when connections between the skin and the spinal cord are first made in the fetus (Bradley & Mistretta 1975), and have also been used to study the postnatal maturation of descending motor pathways (Issler & Stephens 1983). The cutaneous flexor reflex has been shown to be particularly well correlated with sensory input (Woolf 1986). This reflex is evoked only by noxious skin stimulation in adults and acts as a defence mechanism whereby the limb is withdrawn from the offending stimulus (Sherrington 1989). Fitzgerald and colleagues (1988) recently examined the cutaneous flexor reflex thresholds in human infants. Testing was performed using Von Frey hairs (a series of hairs of different diameters and flexibility that are used to assess tactile perception or response to such stimulus). These were applied to the lateral plantar surface of the foot. Following painful stimulus (routine heel lancing), the researchers were able to examine the responses of preterm infants to nociceptive stimulation.

Flexion reflex thresholds in newborn infants are reported to be very low and gradually increase with postconceptual age. The gradual increase of the threshold is not related to postnatal age in premature infants but only to post-conceptual age. Thus, a baby born at 28 weeks gestation and tested four weeks later at 32 weeks will have a similar threshold to a newborn baby born at 32 weeks gestation (Fitzgerald *et al* 1988). These findings, which indicated a hypersensitivity to tissue damage (heel lance) analogous to tenderness or hyperalgesia in adults, suggested that the low thresholds were not directly related to preterm birth itself but rather a feature of the developing reflex. As well as finding low reflex thresholds and increased sensitivity of preterm infants to pain, Fitzgerald and colleagues also found evidence to suggest that repeated handling may result in excessive excitation of central neurones which could affect their function as well as contribute to irregularities in blood pressure. This could have important implications for neonatal nurses and midwives.

□ The role of endogenous opiates

Endogenous opiates (naturally produced morphine-like substances) are released in the human fetus at birth and in response to fetal and neonatal distress (Gautray *et al* 1977). Healthy full term infants who have been delivered normally or by caesarean section have been found to have significantly higher plasma levels of one such opiate, β endorphin, than those found in resting adults. In addition, infants delivered vaginally by breech presentation or by vacuum extraction were found to have further increases in β endorphin levels indicating β endorphin secretion in response to stress at birth (Puolakka *et al* 1982). Levels of β endorphin, over and above those expected for a newborn, have been found in infants with apnoea of prematurity (MacDonald *et al* 1986), infections and hypoxaemia (Hindmarsh & Sankaran 1984).

These elevated levels may have been caused by the stress of illness, the pain associated with these clinical conditions or the invasive procedures required for their treatment (Anand & Hickey 1987). Such high levels of β endorphins, however, are unlikely to decrease anaesthesia or analgesia requirements; the cerebrospinal fluid levels of β endorphins required to produce analgesia in human adults have been found to be 10 000 times higher than the highest recorded levels in neonates (Foley *et al* 1979).

■ The assessment of infant pain

The assessment of infant pain is particularly complex. Tiny babies cannot tell us what they are feeling; they have no language to express the intensity of their hurt. Meeting the needs of the infant in pain requires a systematic, multi-dimensional approach from health professionals. The role of the neonatal nurse and midwife is crucial in interpreting the physiological and behavioural signs which suggest that an infant may be experiencing pain and meeting the need for analgesia must be seen as a dynamic process which must constantly be reviewed and reappraised. Additionally, nurses and midwives should be aware that, while overt illness or acute trauma will produce distinct physiological and behavioural reactions in an infant, there are features of the intensive care environment itself which may add to the overall distress the baby may experience.

□ Environmental and iatrogenic considerations

Many factors require consideration for the appropriate assessment and management of infant pain. In addition to the presence of critical illness and acute tissue damage (as may be caused by the insertion of a drain for example) there are features of the neonatal intensive care unit environment which warrant attention in any discussion of infant pain. The following factors may exacerbate the pain an infant may be experiencing.

- *Noise pollution* has been identified as contributing to major adverse psychophysiological effects in infants. Researchers have reported sleep disturbance, startles, motor arousal and crying, decrease in transcutaneous oxygenation, acceleration of heart rate and increase of intracranial pressure (Long *et al* 1980; Brenig 1982). The latter may have particularly adverse effects as poor autoregulation of haemodynamics and inadequate cerebral blood flow have been found in the most sick and preterm infants who are at high risk for intraventricular haemorrhage (Lou *et al* 1979; Milligan 1980; Friis-Hansen 1985; Greisen 1986).

- *The intensity of light* in neonatal intensive care units has increased five to tenfold over the last two decades (Glass *et al* 1985). The infants in intensive care are frequently exposed to moderate to high light levels 24 hours per day. Infants may be positioned so that they are constantly looking up at bright illumination which may, in itself, contribute to additional physiological distress. Typically, there is no diurnal rhythmicity of light in the NICU, and some investigators believe that this may interfere with the infant's development of normal biological rhythms. Evidence indicates that, under extreme conditions, lighting can have negative biochemical and physical effects on animals and humans (Lawson 1975; Glass 1985; Mann *et al* 1986).

  Until recently, there was no firm evidence that the reported excess of sleep disturbances in preterm infants later in the first year of life (Booth *et al* 1980) could be attributed to an early lack of adequate environmental support in establishing clear diurnal rhythms. A randomised controlled trial by Mann and colleagues (1986), however, confirms the hypothesised beneficial effect of day and night rhythms on the infant. Preterm babies who were cared for in a nursery where the intensity of light and noise was reduced between 7 pm and 7 am spent a significantly longer time sleeping, less time feeding and gained more weight after being discharged home, than those who were nursed in perpetual light and noise. These researchers concluded by referring to the practice in their neonatal unit. 'Our use of constant light' they wrote, 'has evolved from the wish to provide a neonatal unit with an environment that is less stressful and more relaxing to the parents and the staff. The results of this study suggest that it is not in the best longterm interests of the infants or their parents' (Mann *et al* 1986; page 1267).

- *Skin trauma* often results from monitor leads, tape or transcutaneous oxygen monitoring. Preterm infants are particularly susceptible to such trauma.

Appropriate nursing management can contribute significantly to the overall reduction of pain and discomfort suffered by babies in the NICU. This is particularly crucial in cases where systemic analgesia may not be appropriate. There is evidence, however, to suggest that neonatal nurses and midwives may not always be aware of the importance of nursing care in the overall management of infant pain (Fletcher 1990).

☐ **Biochemical responses**

There are limited data available on neonatal responses to venepuncture and other minor procedures. Plasma renin activity increased significantly five times after venepuncture in full term infants and returned to basal levels 60 minutes thereafter. No changes occurred in the plasma levels of cortisol, epinephrine or norepinephrine (hormones often associated with stress) following venepuncture (Fiselier *et al* 1983). In preterm infants receiving ventilation therapy, chest physiotherapy and endotracheal suctioning produced significant increases in plasma epinephrine and norepinephrine. This response was decreased in sedated infants indicating adverse physiological reaction to invasive procedures and handling in the non-sedated group (Greisen *et al* 1985).

Hormonal and metabolic changes have been measured in neonates undergoing surgery. Anand and colleagues (1987) investigated hormonal and metabolic responses to surgery in two groups of preterm infants undergoing ligation of patent ductus arteriosus. One group received 59 per cent nitrous oxide as an anaesthetic while the other received nitrous oxide and Fentanyl (a potent analgesic agent) 10 microgrammes per kg body weight. This study showed significant reduction in adverse effects in the Fentanyl group and suggested there was evidence that the postoperative course of that group was more stable. Adverse effects of surgery under minimal anaesthesia included a marked release of catecholamines, growth hormone, glucogen, cortisol, aldosterone and other corticosteroids, as well as suppression of insulin secretion. These responses resulted in the breakdown of carbohydrate and precious fat stores leading to severe and prolonged hyperglycaemia. Increased protein breakdown was documented in the group receiving minimal anaesthesia both during and after surgery (Anand *et al* 1987). There were felt to be some omissions in their paper (Editorial, *Lancet* 1987). No record of intraoperative blood pressures was provided – values which it is argued would have provided a more reliable indication of level of anaesthesia than heart rate. In addition, no mention was made as to whether the two groups were matched for severity of illness. Nevertheless, these researchers highlighted the plight of infants who may suffer significant and profound physiological disturbance as a direct result of inadequate anaesthesia and analgesia during surgery. No mention is made of the psychological impact of inadequate analgesia on these infants which, it may be postulated, must also have been significant, irrespective of gestation and regardless of their ability to verbalise their experiences.

Changes in plasma stress hormones (cortisol for example) can also be correlated with the behavioural states of newborn infants (Anders *et al* 1970; Tennes & Carter 1973; Gunnar *et al* 1981) which are important in the identification and recognition of overt distress in neonates responding to pain (Anand & Hickey 1987).

The adverse biochemical sequelae of inadequate analgesia during and following surgery, have been described. The neonatal nurse or midwife does not have at her disposal the sophisticated laboratory techniques necessary to detect subtle changes in an infant's biochemistry suggestive of pain. A variety of measures are available, however, to aid the clinician in the assessment of infant pain.

□ **Physiological responses**

Alterations in physiological parameters are routinely monitored in sick neonates. Heart rate, respiratory rate and alteration in blood pressure have been found to vary in response to pain. These physiological reactions indicate the activation of the sympathetic nervous system. Beyer and Byers (1985) suggest, however, that nurses and midwives can neither infer pain from signs of autonomic arousal nor rule out pain in the absence of autonomic arousal. In other words, physiological parameters alone cannot determine whether or not an infant is in pain. In conjunction with other observations, however, physiological parameters can provide useful information in the assessment of infant pain.

Behavioural and physiological responses that communicate pain in humans may be categorised in the following ways (Hester 1979).

1. *Visceral changes* shift the blood supply from organs immediately essential to muscular exertion resulting in increased cardiac output, tachycardia, tachypnoea, pallor, changes in oxygenation, dilated pupils, raised hairs, trembling and perspiration.

2. *Verbal statements*: children under two years are usually unable to convey their thoughts and feelings in language. However, there is evidence to suggest the 'pain cries' of babies may be clearly identified as such by untrained adults (Porter *et al* 1986).

3. *Vocalisation*: crying, groaning, whimpering, grunting, whining, sobbing, screaming or gasping.

4. *Facial expression*: clenched teeth, tightened lips, grimacing, frowning, widening or tightly shutting the eyes, wrinkling the forehead, frowning, clenching the jaws.

5. *Increase or decrease in body activity*: rigid stillness, flailing, kicking, turning, covering the threatened area, twisting or jerking.

6. *Responses to surrounding environments*: pain tends to draw attention to itself and narrows perception (Stewart 1977).

Transcutaneous oxygen pressure and emotional sweating have been studied as psychological responses to stress or pain in the neonate. Rawlings and colleagues (1980) found that transcutaneous oxygen levels in healthy neonates decreased during circumcision and remained low throughout the procedure.

Harpin and Rutter (1982) investigated the development of emotional sweating in newborn infants as an index for the assessment of emotional state of newborn infants. The researchers studied 124 infants of gestational ages 25–41 weeks. Palmar water loss was studied in infants undergoing heel prick for routine blood sampling. In babies of 37 weeks or more gestation, there was a clear relationship between palmar water loss and arousal from the day of birth and, by the third week, levels of vigorous crying indicated a response comparable to that of an anxious adult. (Less mature infants did not show emotional sweating at birth; it was first seen at the equivalent of 36–37 weeks of maturity.) The researchers suggested emotional sweating could be a useful tool for the assessment of emotional state of the newborn (Harpin & Rutter 1982).

Finally, transcutaneous oxygen levels have been shown to increase following vigorous crying (Rawlings *et al* 1980) as a direct consequence of the infant experiencing acute pain. However, during episodes of crying, oxygen delivery to cerebral tissues may be compromised even though the oxygen content of the blood remains stable (Brazy 1988).

Despite such apparent contradictions, monitoring trends of physiological parameters can provide useful information for documenting and evaluating pain in neonates (Frank 1987). There is a continued need for constant observation of sick infants by skilled and experienced neonatal nurses and midwives who recognise behavioural cues of distress in infants.

☐ **Behavioural responses**

Predictable patterns of behaviour have been observed in healthy infants in response to pain and could be useful as indicators of pain in clinical settings. Behavioural assessment of infant pain includes vocalisation (an infant's cry), facial expression and gross motor movement.

Facial expression
In the late 1800s, Darwin first described the facial expression of pain in infants. He described a face that had eyes firmly closed so that the skin around them was wrinkled and the forehead was contracted into a frown. The mouth widely open with the lips retracted in a peculiar manner which

caused it to assume a squarish form, the gums and teeth being more or less exposed.

Following on from Darwin, Izard and colleagues (1983) described facial expressions of infants experiencing pain and observed three areas of the face (brow, eyes and mouth) suggestive of discrete emotional expressions. These included pain, anger, fear, surprise and joy. Expressions of pain included lowered eyebrows drawn together producing a distinct bulge or frown, eyes tightly closed and an angular squarish mouth produced by clenching the jaws together.

More recently, Grunau and Craig (1987) have described discrete facial action and cry in response to painful stimulus. Pain expression in neonates instigated by heel lance for blood sampling purposes was systematically described using measures of facial expression and cry. The authors identified facial expressions similar to those previously described by Izard. Following heel lance, neonates early in the second day of life, showed a constellation of facial changes, namely, vertical furrow above and between the brow occurring as a result of the lowering and drawing together of the eyebrows, taut tongue and open mouth, together with cry response that differed substantially from the amount and type of facial action provoked by heel rub. They described this reaction pattern as 'pain' expression, but suggested that other factors such as the behavioural state of the infant, (whether awake, quiet or crying), temperamental variations or extrinsic variables such as soothing or swaddling during the stimulation may also affect pain behaviour.

In the absence of crying in the case of an intubated infant, the infant has been identified as forming a 'cry face' characteristic of pain (Izard *et al* 1983; Johnstone & Strada 1986).

Cries
Cries associated with pain have been found to be distinct from other cries and can be distinguished accurately by untrained adults (Porter *et al* 1986). Neonatal nurses, midwives and parents have been able to distinguish cries of pain, hunger and fussiness. Specifically the infant in pain has been described as producing an atypical high pitched cry (Zeskind & Lester 1978; Lester & Zeskind 1979; Lester & Zeskind 1982; Golub 1982; Zeskind 1985). Infant studies in the past two decades have shown newborns and infants to have a far greater degree of neurological competence and behavioural organisation than previously believed (Branson 1982; Stratton 1982).

Body movements
Early studies of the motor response of newborn infants to pin pricks reported that infants responded with a disorganised body movement rather than a purposeful withdrawal of the limb (McGraw 1941). In the first ten days following birth, neonates' response to pain (pin prick) was described as general diffuse movements which became more intense in the first month.

By six months of age, the infants were said to exhibit a purposeful with-drawal of the affected limb. By the age of one year infants were reported to touch or rub the painful area. More recently, researchers have found reflex withdrawals to be the most common response (Lipsit & Levy 1959). Motor responses of healthy full term infants to a pin prick on the leg were reported to be flexion and adduction of the upper and lower limbs associated with grimacing, crying or both (Rich *et al* 1974). Frank (1986) has described a study which quantitatively describes pain behaviour in infants. Techniques used to record the responses of ten newborn infants to heelstick procedures at four weeks of age were as follows. Neonates were placed in a warmed cot and video recorded. Latency and velocity of movements were measured with a calibrated grid on the playback monitor screen. The responses con-sisted of an immediate withdrawal of both the affected and unaffected leg, followed by facial grimacing and crying. The results suggested that greater velocity of movements may reflect a greater intensity of pain. Other studies that did not utilise such precise measurements may have missed this import-ant finding.

Recently Cote and colleagues (1991) have systematically examined the behaviours suggestive of pain in four newborn full term infants following major surgery. A case study approach was used and the infants were video taped for 12 hours continuously commencing 24 hours after surgery. The infants' heart rates and respiratory rates were monitored continuously. In addition, their facial expressions, body postures and movements were coded minute by minute from videotapes. The infants were given varying amounts of postoperative analgesia. (The authors note that there was no control over the type of anaesthesia given or over the postoperative regime for admini-stering analgesia.)

The behavioural indices of acute pain were validated by correlating the behaviours demonstrated during infant care that might be considered pain-ful, for example, chest physiotherapy. Episodes of acute pain were evident when the infant was receiving a heelstick, being suctioned or having his position changed. Infants exhibited acute distress by frowning, drawing up their knees and crying. All these infant behaviours were previously validated as being indicative of acute pain (Johnston & Strada 1986; Grunau & Craig 1987).

The infant who received least analgesia demonstrated greater post-operative distress evidenced by his behaviour – which included disrupted sleep patterns, restlessness and posturing (holding his limbs and body taut, drawing his knees to his abdomen). Comparisons of behavioural states (i.e. whether the infant was lying quiet, alert, drowsy, sleeping, experiencing acute distress or crying, before and after analgesia administration, revealed a reduction in crying after administration of analgesia. An important finding was the extent to which analysis of the facial coding system (based on Izard 1983) showed a significant reduction in frowning following the administra-tion of analgesia. Observational analysis of the infants' behaviours showed that brief periods of acute distress also occurred in response to external stimuli such as a loud noise. This frequently occurred when alarms sounded or the lids on rubbish bins slammed. This finding was of concern to the researchers who suggested simple environmental modifications could minimise the distress of infants in general. In addition, despite the extensive handling of the infants by neonatal nurses and midwives, there was relatively little handling of the infants to caress or console them.

Although this study was small, it extends our knowledge and understanding in the area of neonatal pain. In addition to the requirements of infants for systemic analgesia, the study highlights areas of nursing behaviour (for example, decreasing noise levels and providing comforting physical contact where possible) which may contribute to the non-pharmacological treatment of pain and discomfort in infants.

Research into infants' responses to pain have shown that the responses are not uniform or simple. The variety of reactions exhibited by an individual infant are dependent on the infant's gestational age and neurological integrity. In addition, it has been suggested the environment of the NICU may cause an infant additional stress.

■ Infant state regulation

Awareness of the normal maturational process of premature and term infants is useful when assessing pain. Behavioural state describes the behavioural responses of an infant at any given time and is dependent on factors such as gestational age, neurodevelopmental status and the clinical condition of the infant. The Brazelton neonatal behavioural assessment scale (see Fig. 8.1) has been used to monitor behavioural changes in infants undergoing painful procedures (Marshall *et al* 1980). Briefly, infant state regulation is the extent to which the infant can exert control over his

Figure 8.1 The Brazelton neonatal behavioural assessment scale (adapted from Brazelton 1977)

Infant state is defined in six stages:

* Deep sleep
* Light sleep
* Drowsiness
* Quiet alertness
* Fussiness
* Crying

environment. Brazelton's system, which defines infant state in six stages, looks particularly at those infant capabilities which are most important to developing social relationships. For example, how easy is it to console the baby, how quickly does the baby react to various types of stimulation and how quickly does he calm down. Very premature infants may not be able to adapt to their environment as easily as term infants (Amiel-Tison 1985).

Awareness of the nature of an infant's behavioural state may assist the neonatal nurse and midwife with consoling an infant during a painful procedure and in settling the infant following the procedure. For example, comforting, soothing and distracting techniques such as swaddling, rocking and patting (Brazelton 1977; Field & Goldson 1984) have been suggested to provide a calming effect on the infant experiencing pain. Although these strategies have a physiological basis (for example, swaddling reduces irregular movement of the infant), they may have limited use with an infant in an incubator. Nevertheless, gentle containment of an infant's limbs during a painful procedure will reduce irregular movement (flailing of the arms and legs).

Behavioural state has been identified as a powerful indicator as to the effects of the environment on the infant and his ability to interact with his immediate environment, leading to increased or decreased overall distress (Lawhon 1986; Weibley 1989).

In the NICU, pain behaviours may be interpreted as irritability or restlessness. Under these circumstances neonates may be sedated with pharmacological agents such as chloral hydrate or paralysed with drugs such as Pavulon. Neither of these agents is effective in reducing pain perception; however, these drugs can mask pain behaviours of the neonate and may even serve to facilitate the denial of health professionals about how much pain the infant really experiences (Broome & Tanzillo 1990).

Irritability and pain, both of which may be treated to some level with analgesics, are related but distinct phenomena. Each is associated with a different set of behaviours and intervention strategies. Astute clinical judgements made by the neonatal nurse and midwife, based on a comprehensive assessment of the neonate and the environment, will assist in the nursing assessment of neonatal pain. Full term infants who are obviously more neurologically mature than preterm infants, pass their time in varying states of consciousness. According to Brazelton (1973), such states occur cyclically moving from deep sleep to light sleep, from drowsiness to quiet alertness, from fussing to crying and from alertness to drowsiness and back to deep sleep again. Sick or immature infants may not have the ability to regulate their patterns of behaviour and may be assisted to do so by the reflective practitioner who may institute soothing techniques appropriate to the infant's gestation and general condition. For example, non-nutritive sucking, facilitated by use of a pacifier, may comfort and soothe. Infants have been noted to use self-consoling behaviours such as sucking on their own hands

(Brazelton 1973). The smallest preterm infant may be observed to suck on an endotracheal tube.

It is important for neonatal nurses and midwives to remember when considering infant pain that infants' responses to a painful stimulus may not be immediate. The infant may appear to tolerate one or several procedures and then exhibit signs of compromise with increased oxygen requirements in the absence of further stimulation (High & Gorski 1985). This has particular relevance for the very low birthweight infant or the extremely stressed infant. There may be no response at all to noxious stimuli. The immature central nervous system has a limited ability to withstand stress and the absence of response may only indicate the depletion of response capability and not the lack of perception (Frank 1989).

■ Conclusions

Research reports now provide empirical evidence to confirm our suspicions that infants are capable of responding to pain. An important nursing issue is to determine what are the best indicators of neonatal pain and how health care professionals can best recognise them.

The assessment and alleviation of infants' pain may be complicated by the practitioner's inability to give priority to pain management. The abstract and elusive nature of pain may cause this aspect of care to be superseded by other more concrete problems such as fluid and electrolyte balance. Neonatal nurse education programmes currently place minimal emphasis on the knowledge of pain. In addition, research (Frank 1987; Fletcher 1990) has found a lack of consistency in attitudes and practices among staff in neonatal intensive care units; lack of knowledge leading to inadequate assessment and subsequent management of pain has been identified in these studies.

Neonatal nurses and midwives must demonstrate that non-pharmacological comfort measures have been implemented prior to considering systemic analgesia. Systemic analgesia should be used judiciously because the long term effects of these drugs on the developing central nervous system are as yet undetermined (Frank 1989).

Neonatal nurses and midwives need to retain not only the vocabulary of blood gasses, but also the vocabulary of nesting. This, involving the provision of soft bedding for an infant who may be lying naked in an incubator, is used to give the sensation of boundaries to the infant so that his body and limbs are gently contained in a position of flexion, as they were in the womb, in an attempt to increase the infant's sense of security and comfort. Self-containment promotes quietening and self-control and may reduce the overall stress of being nursed in NICU (Fletcher 1990).

■ **Recommendations for clinical practice in the light of currently available evidence**

1. There should be ongoing discussion, collaboration and agreement between medical and nursing/midwifery staff regarding the efficacy and provision of local and systemic analgesia for a variety of procedures and conditions (Fletcher 1990). The emotional and psychological aspects of neonatal nursing must not be eclipsed by the aggressive medical model of care.

2. Neonatal nurses and midwives must consider present routine care (such as the automatic changing of nappies every three or four hours) in the light of the proven relationship between adverse physiological disruption and excessive handling.

3. The success of individualised care minimising the effects of the NICU environment on infants is, however, dependent on carers' knowledge of specific environmental factors and their potential for harm. Managers must take responsibility, therefore, for arranging in-service education and the provision of current and topical reading material for nurses and midwives working in such specialist areas as neonatal intensive care.

4. As neonatal nurses and midwives increase their technical knowledge and skills in pain management, they can help to counteract ignorance and challenge established, but mistaken, modes of thinking.

5. Neonatal nurses and midwives must be stronger advocates for their patients and their families. There are many aspects of the NICU environment which could be changed. For example, levels of noise and light could be reduced; activities could be 'clustered' so that periods of restful sleep can be experienced by sick infants.

6. The importance of comfort and a friendly environment should not be underestimated. Infants respond to stimuli such as touch, trauma, light and noise, and may be aware of more than we yet realise.

7. Respect for persons through respect for autonomy includes all patients who can communicate. Newborns' responses to all caregiving procedures, from the provision of nesting to the insertion of chest drains, must be viewed and interpreted as expressions of assent or dissent rather than as mere behaviours (Cunningham 1990). All caregivers can promote infant autonomy by learning 'the language of attentive patient care' as it may apply to infants (Mishler *et al* 1989).

■ Practice check

- Consider an infant in your care.

- Is an obvious pain stimulus present, such as a chest or abdominal drain? Has the infant been recently intubated? Are there signs of extravasation?

- Have the infant's care taking activities been grouped to allow minimal disturbance?

- What non-pharmacological comfort measures have been promoted (for example, nesting, non-nutritive sucking)?

- What does the infant look like? Are infant responses related to position changes, feeding schedules or rest times?

- Is it always borne in mind in your unit that the babies receiving care are people (who can experience sensation) and not objects? What kinds of descriptions are given of the infants on rounds and what kind of entries are put into charts? Do caregivers remember and use the baby's correct name and sex?

- Are there decorations on incubators and mobiles above them? They help to modify the intensive care environment and spread comfort more than they do infection.

- Are parents greeted warmly and made to feel welcome? Do you make it clear to them that you regard their baby as an individual, while encouraging and supporting them to do the same?

□ Acknowledgement

I would like to thank Mrs Janette Drysdale for her help in typing this manuscript.

■ References

Amiel-Tison C 1985 Paediatric contribution in the present knowledge on the neurobehavioural status of infants at birth. In Mehler J, Fox R (eds) Neonatal cognition: beyond the blooming buzzing confusion. Lawrence Erlbaum, New Jersey

Anand K J S, Hickey P R 1987 Pain and its effects in the human neonate and fetus. New England Journal of Medicine 317 (21): 1321–9

Anand K J S, Sippell W G, Aynsley-Green A 1987 A randomised trial of fentanyl anaesthesia in pre-term neonates undergoing surgery: effects on the stress response. Lancet 1: 243–8

Anders T F, Sachar E J, Krean J, Roffwarg H P, Hellman L 1970 Behavioural state and plasma cortisol response in the human newborn. Paediatrics 46: 532–7

Arduini D, Rizzo G, *et al* 1986 The development of fetal behavioural states: a longitudinal study. Prenatal Diagnosis 6: pp 117–24

Berry F A, Gregory G A 1987 Do premature infants require anaesthesia for surgery? Anaesthesiology 67: 291–3

Beyer J, Byers M L 1985 Knowledge of paediatric pain: state of the art. Children's Health Care 13: 150–59

Booth C L, Lennart H L, Toman E G 1980 Sleep states and behaviour pattern in pre-term and full term infants. Neuropediatrics 11: 354–64

Bradley R M, Mistretta C M 1975 Fetal sensory receptors. Physiology Reviews 55: 352–82

Branson G W 1982 Structures, status and characteristics of the nervous system at birth. In Strattan P (ed) Psychobiology of the human newborn. John Wiley, New York

Brazelton T B 1973 Neonatal behavioural assessment scale. Clinics in Developmental Medicine No 50. Spastics International Medical Publications, London

Brazelton T B 1977 Neonatal behaviour and its significance. In Schaffer A J, Avery M E (eds) Diseases of the newborn. W B Saunders, Philadelphia

Brazy J A 1988 Effects of crying on cerebral blood flow and cytochrome 993. Journal of Paediatrics 112 (3): 457–61

Brenig F A 1982 Infant incubator study. Dissertation for the Degree of Doctor of Public Health, School of Public Health, Faculty of Medicine, Columbia University. Cited in Wolke D 1987 Environmental and developmental neonatology. Journal of Reproductive and Infant Psychology 5: 17–42

Broome M E, Tanzillo H 1990 Differentiating between pain and agitation in premature neonates. Journal of Perinatal and Neonatal Nursing 4 (1): 53–62

Cote J J, Morse J M, James S G 1991 The pain response of the post operative newborn. Journal of Advanced Nursing 16: 378–87

Cunningham N 1990 Ethical perspectives on the perception and treatment of neonate's pain. Journal of Perinatal and Neonatal Nursing 4 (1): 75–83

Darwin C R The expression of emotions in man and animals. Reprinted 1965, University of Chicago Press, New York, London

Field T, Goldson E 1984 Pacifying effects of non-nutritive sucking of term and pre-term neonates during heelstick procedures. Paediatrics 74: 1012–15

Fiselier T, Monnens L, Moerman E, Van Munster P, Jansen M, Peer P 1983 Influence of the stress of venepuncture on basal levels of plasma renin activity in infants and children. International Journal of Paediatric Nephrology 4: 181–5

Fitzgerald M, Millard C, MacIntosh N 1989 Cutaneous hypersensitivity following peripheral tissue damage in newborn infants and its reversal with topical analgesia. Pain 39: 31–6

Fitzgerald M, Shaw A, MacIntosh N 1988 Cutaneous flexor reflex thresholds in human infants. Developmental Medicine and Child Neurology 30 (4): 520–26

Fletcher D V 1990 A study of neonatal nurses' and midwives' perceptions of pain and discomfort in the neonate. Internal Report March 1990. Glasgow Royal Maternity Hospital, Glasgow

Foley K M, Kourides I A, Inturrisi C E, *et al* 1979 β-endotrophin: analgesic and hormonal effects in humans. Proceedings of the National Academy of Science USA 76: 5377–81

Frank L S 1989 Pain in one non-verbal patient: advocating for the critically ill neonate. Paediatric Nursing 15 (1): 65–8, 90

Frank L S 1987 A national survey of the assessment of pain and agitation in the neonatal intensive care unit. Journal of Obstetrics, Gynaecology and Neonatology 16 (6): 387–93

Frank L S 1986 A new method to quantitatively describe pain behaviour in infants. Nursing Research 35: 28–31

Friis-Hansen B 1985 Perinatal brain injury and cerebral blood flow in newborn infants. Acta Paediatrica Scandinavica 74: 323–31

Gautray J P, Jolivet A, Uileh J P, Guillemin R 1977 Immunoassayable β-endotrophin in human amniotic fluid: elevation in cases of fetal distress. American Journal of Obstetrics and Gynecology 129: 211–12

Glass E, Avery G G, Subrananlou K N S, Keys M P, Sostek A M, Friendly D S 1985 Effect of bright light in the hospital nursery on the incidence of retinopathy of prematurity. New England Journal of Medicine 313: 401–4

Gleiss J, Stuttgen G 1970 Morphologic and functional development of the skin. In Stave U (ed) Physiology of the perinatal period, Vol 2. Appleton Century Crofts, New York

Golub H L, Corwin M J 1982 Infant cry: a clue to diagnosis. Paediatrics 69: 197–201

Greisen G 1986 Cerebral blood flow and pre-term infants during the first week of life. Acta Paediatrica Scandinavica 75: 43–51

Greisen G, Frederiksen P S, Hertel J, Christensen N J 1985 Catecholamine response to chest physiotherapy and endotracheal suctioning in pre-term infants. Acta Paediatrica Scandinavica 74: 525–9

Grunau R V E, Craig K D 1987 Pain expression in neonates: facial action and cry. Pain 28: 395–410

Gunnar M R, Fisch R O, Kirsvik S, Donohowe J M 1981 The effects of circumcision on serum cortisol and behaviour. Psychoneuroendocrinology 6: 269–75

Harpin V A, Rutter N 1982 Development of emotional sweating in the newborn infant. Archives of Disease in Childhood 57: 691–5

Henderson-Smart D J, Pettigrew A G, Campbell D J 1983 Clinical apnoea and brain stem neural function in pre-term infants. New England Journal of Medicine 7: 308–53

Hester N K 1979 The pre-operational child's reaction to immunization. Nursing Research 28: 250–51

High A, Gorski P 1985 Recording environmental influences on infant development in the ICU: womb for improvement. In Gottfried A, Gaiter J L (eds) Infant's stress under intensive care. University Park Press, Baltimore

Hindmarsh K W, Sankaran K 1984 Endorphins and the neonate. Canadian Medical Association Journal 132: 331–4

Issler H, Stephens J A 1983 The maturation of cutaneous reflexes studied in the upper limb in man. Journal of Physiology 335: 643–54

Izard C E, Hembree E A, Dougherty Y L, Spizarri M 1983 Changes in facial expression of 2 to 19 month old infants following acute pain. Developmental Psychology 19 (3): 418–26

Janko M, Trantel J 1983 Flexion withdrawal reflex as recorded from single human biceps femoris motor neurones. Pain 15: 167–76

Johnstone C C, Strada M E 1986 Acute pain response in infants: a multiple dimensional description. Pain 24: 373–82

Lancet 1987 Editorial: Pain anaesthesia and babies. Lancet ii: 543–4

Lawhon G 1986 Management of stress in premature infants. In Angelini D J, Whelan-Knapp C K, Gibes R M (eds) Perinatal/neonatal nursing: a clinical handbook. Blackwell Scientific Press, Boston

Lawson K, Darwin C, Turkewitz G 1977 The environmental characteristics of a NICU. Child Development 48: 1633–9

Lester B M, Zeskind P S 1982 A behavioural perspective on crying in early infancy. In Fitzgerald H E, Lester B M, Wogman M W (eds) Theory and research and behavioural paediatrics, Vol 1. Plenum, New York

Lipsit C P, Levy N 1959 Electroactual threshold in the neonate. Child Development 30: 547–54

Long G J, Lucey J F, Philip A G S 1980 Noise and hypoxaemia in the intensive care nursery. Paediatrics 65: 143–5

Lou H C, Lassen N A, Friis-Hansen B 1979 Impaired auto-regulation of cerebral blood flow and the distressed newborn infant. Journal of Paediatrics 94: 118–21

MacDonald M C G, Moss I R, *et al* 1986 Effect of Naltrexane on apnoea of prematurity and on plasma beta-endorphin-like immunoreactivity. Development in Pharmacology Therapy 9: 301–309

McGraw M B 1941 Neural mechanisms as exemplified in the changing reactions of the infant to pin prick. Child Development 12: 31–41

Mann N P, Haddow R, Stokes L, Goodley S, Rutter N 1986 Effect of night and day on pre-term infants in a newborn nursery: randomized trial. British Medical Journal 293: 1265–7

Marshall R E, Straiton W C, Moore J A, Boxerman S B 1980 Circumcision: effects on newborn behaviour. Infant Behaviour Development 3 (2): 1–14

Milligan P W A 1980 Failure of auto-regulation and intraventricular haemorrhage in pre-term infants. Lancet i: 896–8

Mishler E G, Clark J A, Ingeltinger J 1989 The language of attentive patient care: a comparison of two medical interviews. Journal of General International Medicine 4: 425–35

Owens M E 1984 Pain in infancy: conceptual and methodological issues. Pain 20: 213–30

Porter F L, Porges S E, Miller R H, Marshall R E 1986 Newborn cries and vagal tone: parallel changes in response to circumcision. Child Development 57: 790–802

Puolakka J, Kauppila A, Leppaluoto J, Vuolteenano O 1982 Elevated beta-endorphin immunoreactivity in umbilical cord blood after complicated delivery. Acta Obstetrica Gynaecologica Scandinavica 61: 513–14

Rawlings D J, Miller P A, Engel R R 1980 The effect of circumcision on transcutaneous PO_2 in term infants. American Journal of Disease in Childhood 134: 676–8

Rich E C, Marshall R E, Volpe J J 1974 The normal neonatal response to pin prick. Development in Medicine and Child Neurology   16: 432–4

Schulte F J 1975 Neurophysiological aspects of brain development. Mead Johnstone Symposium in Perinatal Development   6: 38–47

Sherrington C S 1989 Experiments in the examination of the peripheral distribution of the fibres of the posterious roots of some spinal nerves. Part 2: Philosophical transactions of The Royal Society of London, series B. A (190): 45–186

Spehlmann R 1981 EEG primer. Elsevier/North Holland, New York: 159–65

Stewart M C 1977 Measurement of pain. In Jacox A K (ed) Pain: a source book for nurses and other health professionals. Little Brown, Boston

Stratton P 1982 Rhythmic functions in the newborn. In Stratton P (ed) Psychobiology of the human newborn. John Wiley, New York

Tennes K, Carter D 1973 Plasma cortisol levels and behavioural states in early infancy. Psychosomatic Medicine   35: 121–8

Torres F, Anderson C 1985 The normal EEG of the human newborn. Journal of Clinical Neurophysiology   2: 89–103

Wall P D, Melzack R (eds) 1984 The textbook of pain. Churchill Livingstone, Edinburgh

Weibley T T 1989 Inside the incubator. The American Journal of Maternal and Child Nursing   14 (2): 96–100

Woolf C J 1986 Functional plasticity of the flexion withdrawal reflex in the rat following peripheral tissue injury. Advances in Pain Research Therapy   9: 193–210

Zeskind P S 1985 A developmental perspective of infant crying. In Barry M, Lester B M, Zachariah Bourkydis C F (eds) Infant crying: theoretical and research perspectives

Zeskind P S, Lester B M 1978 Acoustic features and auditory perception of the cries of newborns with prenatal and perinatal complications. Child Development   49: 580–89

■ Suggested further reading

Holmes D L, Reich J N, Pasternak J F (eds) 1984 The development of infants born at risk. Lawrence Erlbaum, London, New Jersey

Gaiter J L 1985 Nursery environments. In Gottfried A W, Gaiter J L (eds) Environmental Neonatology. University Park Press, Baltimore

Lawhon G 1986 Management of stress in premature infants. In Angelini D J, Whelan-Knapp C K, Gibes R M (eds) Perinatal/neonatal nursing: a clinical handbook. Blackwell Scientific Press, Boston

Chapter 9

Workload measurement in midwifery

Jean A. Ball

> Tell the computer how sick the patients are and it will tell you how many nurses they need
>
> Jelinek *et al* 1973

The primary purpose for workload research is to assess the volume and variety of demands which groups of patients make upon nursing/midwifery time and skill, in order to provide the number and mix of staff needed to provide a satisfactory standard of care, and to do so in an efficient manner.

During the last 20 years a number of studies have sought to define and measure nursing workload. Most of these studies have been in general nursing. This chapter will review the methods used in these studies, and the work in midwifery which is now emerging.

Throughout this chapter numerous studies on workload will be discussed. Most of these were undertaken in nursing rather than midwifery, some concerned mixed groups of clients/patients. The terms 'patient' and 'nurse' will be used where this is specific to the study in hand, or where these were the terms used by the original author of the study.

■ **It is assumed that you are already familiar with the following terms:**

• Whole time equivalents, staff in post, staffing establishments, direct and indirect care of patients, administrative work, associated work, non-nursing work.

■ **What do we mean by 'workload'?**

The notion of measuring workload first began in manufacturing industry. Production line workers deal with inanimate objects, and the components

154

being tooled by a machine are standard in size, shape and consistency. This is not the case with health care, where individual patients and clients have individual needs. Gillies (1982) quotes a study carried out at the Johns Hopkins Hospital which showed that nursing workload has two main components; one that is fairly constant across all service units (mainly indirect care and administration) and another which varies with the number and type of patients and is related to their direct care needs. Recognising this variability in patients' needs is an important issue in designing workload research methods.

Implied in most of the workload literature is a view which may be summarised thus:

> Nursing workload consists of the work required to meet the needs of the patients in a particular place and time, plus other activities needed for the planning, review, organisation and support of that care.

Although such a definition appears to be relatively simple, it hides a complex and constantly changing picture. Many factors affect nursing workload patterns; the numbers and case mix of patients, the degree of emergency or unplanned admissions, the work patterns of doctors, the demands of student training, etc. In a recent report, the Audit Commission (1991) recounts its surprise at the many factors which impinge on the planning and delivery of patient care.

In seeking to produce measures of workload certain issues must be addressed.

1. The need for valid assessment of the variety and volume of patients' needs, in different wards and at different times
Studies which have simply divided the nursing hours available by the number of patients have either made unfounded assumptions about the efficiency of nursing allocation (National Audit Office 1985) or have pointed out the difficulty of drawing conclusions in the absence of more sensitive workload information. One such is the study by Reid and Melaugh (1988) which compared the nurse hours per patient day allocated in 45 different midwifery wards in Northern Ireland. The results showed a clear variation in nurse hours per patient day in wards of a similar size, but as no method for measuring patient dependency was used it was not possible to explain these variations in staff allocation. The authors assume with some justification, that the differences were due to the routine allocation of staff to wards in different hospitals. Their study raises a number of important questions as to the rationale behind nurse or midwife allocation.

2. Making allowances for other demands upon staff time
Several studies have shown nursing time being used for activities such as clerical, portering, and domestic work due to the lack of support staff in a

ward (Ball & Oreschnik 1986b; Gillett & Flux 1987; Hilton & Dawson 1988; Ball *et al* 1989).

3. Questions of quality

This is a dilemma which faces all researchers in this field. One of the major difficulties in undertaking measures of patient/nursing workload is to determine whether the time being spent on an item of patient care equals the time needed to give a satisfactory standard of care. When observing nursing activity, one can only observe and record time that is available from staff allocated to the ward at that time, and this may be more or less than that needed.

This was an issue faced by Senior (1979). Using a dependency based approach for observation of nursing time, she overcame the problem by making ample staff available on the wards during the time of observation, and preventing the withdrawal of allocated staff to other wards or activities. She also asked the ward sister to indicate the degree to which she considered that good nursing care had been given. On this premise therefore, Senior considered that 'real' nursing time needed could be demonstrated, although her study was criticised because of the subjective nature of the assessment of satisfactory care. Ball and Goldstone (1984) addressed this issue by incorporating an independent audit tool (Monitor – Goldstone *et al* 1983) into a dependency based workload system.

■ Basic principles and approaches to measuring workload

A review of the literature reveals two main approaches to measuring workload, the dependency based approach and the identification of 'standard times'.

☐ Dependency based

This method uses some form of classifying patients into different categories of need for nursing attention, and measures the time per day required to meet the different categories of dependence, by observing and recording actual nursing time spent on direct care (Barr 1967; Barr *et al* 1973; Rhys Hearn 1974; Ball & Goldstone 1984).

☐ Standard times for nursing tasks per patient

This approach identifies the direct care nursing interventions or tasks required by different patients, and assesses the average time needed to perform each activity, either by observation or consensus estimation (Auld 1976; Bell & Storey 1984).

Both approaches result in calculating the number of nursing hours required by patient workload, the differences in approach being mainly philosophical. Most workload studies also examine the nursing time required for indirect care and other duties and add this to the time required per patient.

A further approach used for estimating the staff needed in intensive and special care units has been to use clinical indicators of a patient's condition and to make arbitrary but professionally justifiable calculations of the number of nurses per patient or cot per shift required to provide optimum care.

■ Research in nursing/midwifery workload systems

Much of this research was pioneered in the United States where the need to accurately cost nursing care as part of hospital billing of insurance companies created the need for workload measurement. Information from nursing workload systems was then used to underpin nursing organisation and decision making (Gillies 1982; Giovannetti 1984).

In the United Kingdom, workload research began in the 1970s. At this time, staffing guidelines were set by Regional Health Authorities who recommended the number of staff per bed (top down methods) rather than by patient based measurements of need (bottom up methods) (DHSS 1983). Many of the earlier studies were carried out to help Regional Health authorities in this task.

□ Major studies in workload assessment

With the exception of Auld (1976), the majority of nursing workload research was primarily concerned with general nursing care. Most of the studies were carried out by operational research officers or statisticians (Goddard 1963; SSHD 1969; Barr & Moores 1972) or by nurses undertaking academic research (Rhys Hearn 1974; Auld 1976; Lelean 1976; Grant 1979). With the exception of the Aberdeen formula (SHHD 1969) the studies were not repeated over time in order to assess changes in workload which might require changes to be made in the number of staff required.

The study by Auld is notable because it was carried out in maternity care. She studied patients/clients in five groups according to the kind of care they were receiving: inpatient antenatal care, termination of pregnancy, intrapartum care, postnatal and neonatal care. For each of these groups a master sheet containing a list of the nursing activities needed by patients in each group was devised. By observation of staff caring for patients, the *average* time for each activity was assessed. Thus Auld used a standard time per activity approach. The results were then used to build up a picture of the time needed per annum for the number of patients receiving care in the hospital, and by applying the total time needed to the number of patients in each category, a staffing establishment could be produced. Auld added calculation of time needed for teaching student midwives, and provided a method for assessing the skill mix required to match patient need by recommending percentages of time for different grades and types of staff. This was a very robust, forward looking study which sadly has been largely ignored by midwifery services as a whole.

The work by Barr (1967, 1973, 1984) was fundamental in developing a dependency based approach. His studies classified patients into five groups from self-care, intermediate 1 and 2, intermediate bedfast and intensive care. Workload ratios were given to the patients in the different groups which reflected the increasing need for nursing attention. Thus by multiplying the number of patients in each group by the workload ratios for each group a weighted score could be obtained which indicated the ward workload index.

> **E.g.** 5 group 1 patient = 5 (self-care)
> 4 group 2 patients = 4 × 2 = 8 (intermediate 1)
> 5 group 3 patients = 5 × 3 = 15 (intermediate 2)
> 3 group 4 patients = 3 × 4 = 12 (intermediate bedfast)
> 2 group 5 patients = 2 × 5 = 10 (intensive care)
> Ward workload = 5 + 8 + 15 + 12 + 10 = 50
> *Nineteen patients = workload of 50 if they are in the groups shown*

However if the mix was 19 patients distributed as shown below, then the workload index would be different.

> **E.g.** 7 group 1 patients = 7
> 4 group 2 patients = 4 × 2 = 8
> 6 group 3 patients = 18
> 1 group 4 patients = 4
> 1 group 5 patients = 5
> *Ward workload* = 7 + 8 + 18 + 4 + 5 = 42

It is easy to see how workload indices can be used to show changes in workload over time.

□ Current nursing workload sytems

Most of the earlier studies were used to set nursing establishments and information gathering ceased once the study was complete. The need to rationalise staffing numbers and the impact of the Resource Management Initiative has led to the assessment of workload on a daily basis. The resulting data are then used to determine daily and total establishment needs. There are many variations on this theme. Three main approaches will be outlined, Cheltenham, Criteria for Care and Grasp.

Cheltenham (FIP) system (Bell & Storey 1984)

This primarily uses the standard time per activity approach, but a simple patient dependency system is included. Each day, nurses assess the activities needed by the patient to produce the nurse hours per day required. Standard times for activities are calculated by observation and using professional nursing judgement on satisfactory standards of care.

Criteria for Care (Ball et al 1984)

This is a version of the American Rush Medicus System (Jelinek *et al* 1976, 1977) adapted to British practice. Daily dependency assessment using detailed criteria is used to produce workload indices and staff needed (Ball & Oreshnik 1986a, 1986b). The staff time per patient is calculated from the results of a detailed study using non-participant observation. The nursing time spent on the direct patient care of patients in each dependency category is recorded, together with a record of nursing time spent in indirect care, associated work and miscellaneous activities. A quality review using Monitor (Goldstone *et al* 1983) is also carried out. Wards which achieve a predetermined degree of quality are then used as 'model wards', and the nursing patterns in these wards are used to define the nursing time required to cover all patient care and all other nursing activities. Later work added a skill mix assessment (Ball *et al* 1989).

Grasp (Meyer 1984)

This is an American system which combines patient dependency and standard times per activity. A score sheet is completed daily in which different degrees of need for nursing interventions receive predetermined scores which relate to units of nursing time required for each intervention. This builds into a total score per patient which can be used for care planning and calculating total ward workload. The nurse units per score are produced by observation and consensus and are said to reflect agreed standards of patient care.

□ **Assessing workload/staffing in intensive care situations**

A number of attempts have been made to provide guidelines for staffing neonatal units (BPA & RCOG 1977, 1982; Royal College of Physicians 1988), and many of these issues have been reviewed by Pittman (1991). The BPA/RCOG proposals classified neonates into three groups – special care, high dependency and intensive care – recommending minimum numbers of staff per cot as a basis for setting staffing establishments. Although the principles established could have been used to determine neonatal workload over time, they were in fact mainly used by planners. Therefore *cots* were designated as high or low dependency rather than the babies who occupied them. Increases in the number of babies needing intensive care, and the development of new neonatal care techniques meant that a historical staffing establishment could rapidly become out of date (Boxall & Garcia 1983). It would of course be possible for the definitions of need to be used to assess daily workload, and this is how staffing for adult intensive care units is assessed (Intensive Care Society 1985).

In adult intensive care units, patients are classified as low, intermediate or high dependency according to a series of clinical and physiological indicators (Knaus *et al* 1981; Morgan 1986). Nursing levels are set per shift at: two nurses for high dependency, one nurse for intermediate and half a nurse for low dependency patients. Recording the number and mix of patients in each group per shift produces day to day staffing and establishment numbers needed. Ball (1988) used this clinical indicator approach to measure workload in delivery suites.

■ Developments in midwifery practice

Sadly most of the nursing workload literature shows how frequently researchers have sought new paths rather than building on previous research. Midwifery has been somewhat tardy in addressing these issues for itself, and part of the reason has been the reluctance to adopt nursing based systems. Reviewing the literature indicates that there are certain basic principles of workload measurement which can be applied and developed in relation to particular client/patient groups. Birthrate (Ball 1988, 1989, 1992) uses a combination of critical indicator/dependency based approach for measuring workload and outcomes in delivery suites/intrapartum care; while Maclean and Bowden's (1989) system is based upon standard time principles. Both studies are discussed below.

■ Birthrate

Measuring workload during labour and delivery raises a number of research problems:

- The degree of fluctuation on workload on a delivery suite would require observation over a long period of time before a typical pattern could be estimated, and this is very expensive in research time;

- The staff time available might not match the time required by the clients;

- It is difficult to assign women to dependency groups in labour because of the unpredictability of the process or outcome of labour for mother and baby.

Seeking to overcome these problems Ball designed a retrospective assessment of the needs of mother and baby during labour and delivery, based upon clinical indicators. The standard of care and time needed was based upon the recommendations of the Short Report (HC 1980), and the Maternity Care in Action Report (Maternity Services Advisory Committee 1985) both of which recommend that women should have the undivided attention of a midwife throughout labour and delivery. Once this principle has been grasped, the time spent by the mother in the delivery suite from admission to transfer out with her baby becomes the basis for assessing staff time needed. In line with the principles in intensive care units further increases of midwife time are provided for more complicated cases.

Birthrate has three main components:

1. Score system
The midwife completes a score sheet (Fig. 9.1) just before the mother and her baby leave the delivery suite. Each of the indicators has a weighted score designed to reflect the different processes of labour and delivery, and the degree to which these deviated from obstetric normality. The total score is used to allocate the woman and baby to one of five different categories of maternal and neonatal outcome. The lower the score, the more normal are the processes of labour and delivery. Increasing degrees of intervention, crisis or support are reflected in the higher categories. The highest category (V) includes many cases of emergency caesarean section, but also those women who achieve a normal delivery and a healthy baby following high levels of support during labour (e.g. diabetic mothers) or who experience unexpected complications for mother or baby following delivery.

Other categories (X, A and R) are used to identify women who are admitted to the delivery suite for reasons other than labour and delivery. At the present time, this considerable workload is not shown in measures of bed occupancy or the number of deliveries. Provision is also made for estimating workload from flying squads etc.

The number and mix of cases per category produces the individual workload pattern for a particular hospital. Table 9.1 shows the data from 7 hospitals in the Trent Region.

2. Time
The midwife records the length of time spent by the mother in the delivery suite. The mean time in the delivery suite per patient category forms the

Figure 9.1 Birthrate score sheet

Name and address of mother	Date of delivery	
....	Time of delivery	
....		

Section A   Gestation and labour

Gestation	More than 37 weeks	1
	More than 34 weeks, less than 37	2
	Less than 34 weeks	3
Length of	8 hours or less	1
labour	More than 8 hours	2
As required	I.V. infusion (not blood transfusion)	2
	Epidural in situ	3
	Continuous fetal monitoring	3
* *(see note*	Twins*	2
on multiple	Triplets, quadruplets etc*	5
birth scores)	Medical problems needing consultant oversight;	
	e.g. diabetes, heart or chest conditions	5

Subtotal Section A

Section B   Delivery

	Normal delivery	1
	Forceps/breech etc.	2
	Elective Caesarean section	3
	Emergency Caesarean section	5
	Perineum intact	1
	Vaginal/perineal sutures for tear/episiotomy	2
	Extended episiotomy/4th degree tear	3

Subtotal Section B

Section C   Infant(s)

	Apgar score 8+	1
	Apgar score between 5 and 7	2
	Apgar score less than 5	3
	Birth weight 2.5kg or more	1
	Birth weight 1.5kg–2.5kg	2
	Birth weight less than 1.5kg	3
As required	Paediatrician called at or after delivery	2
	Congenital abnormality	3
	Infant is stillborn/dies immediately after birth	5

Subtotal Section C

Section D   Other intensive care

	I.V. infusion given post-delivery	2
	Blood transfusion at any stage	5
	Elective general/spinal anaesthetic	3
	Emergency general/spinal anaesthetic	5
	Intensive care not accounted for by any other factor	5

Subtotal Section D

TOTAL SCORES AND INDICATE CATEGORY AS SHOWN BELOW

Score 6 = Category I	Score 14–18 = Category IV
Score 7–9 = Category II	Score 19+ = Category V
Score 10–13 = Category III	Other categories X A R
Length of time in delivery suite .... hours	

Table 9.1 Numbers and percentage distribution of birthrate outcome measures in seven Trent RHA hospitals over three months

Hospitals		Delivery outcome categories									
	Cat. I		Cat. II		Cat. III		Cat. IV		Cat. V		Total
	N	%	N	%	N	%	N	%	N	%	delivered
A	39	2.5	182	11.6	392	25.0	351	22.4	238	15.2	1202
B	58	4.8	169	14.1	320	26.7	200	1.7	103	8.6	850
C	138	6.1	362	15.9	463	20.3	317	13.9	268	11.8	1548
D	95	9.8	302	31.0	105	10.8	116	11.9	75	7.7	693
E	58	4.4	182	13.8	244	18.5	202	15.3	148	11.3	834
F	94	5.1	264	14.2	362	19.5	342	18.4	288	15.5	1350
G	55	3.2	209	12.3	344	20.2	343	20.2	207	12.2	1158
Total	537	4.9	1670	15.3	2230	20.5	1871	17.2	1327	12.2	7635

Note percentages shown total less than 100 per cent. These data are part of total for all admission of which Table 9.3 (Category X) completes the full data

basis for calculating workload indices and staffing needs. As the more complicated cases require more than one midwife for some of the time, percentages of time are added to the mean time per category, as follows: Category III, 20 per cent; Category IV, 30 per cent; Category V, 40 per cent. An example is shown in Table 9.2 overleaf.

3. Calculating workload and staff needed

Once sufficient data have been collected to calculate the mean average time needed per category, workload indices can be produced and used for calculating the number of midwives needed to provide care to the measured workload. An example is shown below.

Daily workload = daily mean number of cases per category based upon at least six months data multiplied by workload ratios.

	Birthrate Categories				
	I	II	III	IV	V
Mean daily number of cases =	1.7	2.9	1.5	1.2	1.0
multiply by workload ratios =	1	1.34	2.14	2.6	4.2
workload index =		$1.7 + 3.89 + 3.21 + 3.12 + 4.2 = 16.12$			

Multiply the workload index by the time needed for category I (5.9 hours)

= $16.12 \times 5.9 = 95.11$ hours per day for all direct and indirect care. $95.11 \times 7 = 665.76$ hours per week. A further allowance of 15% is added to allow for teaching, management etc.
$665.76 \times 1.15 = 765.62$ hours/37.5 = 20.42 whole time equivalent midwives needed.

To this figure should be added the staff time needed for cases in categories X, A, and R, and a further allowance of 20 per cent for holidays and sickness should also be added to arrive at the total midwife establishment needed.

Table 9.2   Six months Birthrate data January 1–June 30 1991

1.   Number and distribution of Birthrate categories (delivered cases)

Month	I	II	III	IV	V	Total
			Categories			
January	33	78	34	30	40	215
February	28	81	44	33	47	233
March	17	75	45	23	45	205
April	20	64	45	33	35	197
May	15	85	51	29	40	220
June	29	102	34	38	46	249
Totals	142	485	253	186	249	1319
%	10.8	36.9	19.2	14.2	18.9	100
Mean cases per month	23.6	80.83	42.16	31.00	41.5	220

2.   Mean hours in delivery suite January–June 1991

	I	II	III	IV	V
			Category		
January	6.03	7.13	8.21	10.98	16.2
February	5.55	8.2	11.25	10.7	14.3
March	5.57	7.41	10.05	10.9	17.5
April	4.33	6.85	8.9	9.46	18.46
May	5.13	7.91	9.55	12.37	15.0
June	5.44	7.06	8.94	11.25	13.32
Mean	5.34	7.43	9.48	10.93	15.80
% increase	–	–	20	30	40
Midwife hours =	5.9	7.9	12.5	15.3	24.6
Workload ratios	1	1.34	2.14	2.6	4.2

□   **Challenging care policies**

Birthrate data has been used to challenge care practices and to monitor outcomes when care policies have been changed. For example – moving to 24 hour epidural service, allocating low risk women to 'birthing room'. The outcome data can also be used to assess the number of postnatal beds required (Ball 1992).

Table 9.3   Numbers of mothers in Category X (undelivered) shown as percentage of total cases (Trent hospitals) over three months

Hospitals	Category X	% all admissions
A	365	23.4
B	349	29.1
C	728	32.0
D	280	28.8
E	484	36.7
F	508	27.3
G	543	31.9
Total	3257	29.9

Many hospitals have been surprised at the large number of women admitted to delivery suites who are not delivered on their first admission (Category X). Table 9.3 shows that they may account for almost 30 per cent of all admissions.

☐   **Development and validation of Birthrate**

Birthrate (Ball 1988, 1989) was developed at Lincoln County Hospital and validated by blind comparative evaluation of patients' records over six months. Reliability was assessed by regular, random checking of records. Over a six months period, 95 per cent of all score sheets were found to be accurately recorded. The validity and reliability of the method was tested further at three other hospitals in 1986. A further one year study in Trent Region applied Birthrate in three teaching and four non-teaching hospitals.

☐   **The Portsmouth Study**

The Birthrate scoring system formed the basis for a further study of validity and reliability of dependency based criteria for delivery suites (Brown & Dawson 1989). Their study showed, that, contrary to midwives' beliefs, classifying mothers according to different levels of need did show consistent patterns of distribution of time required and given to clients in the different categories. Brown and Dawson extended the workload criteria by defining, more specifically, certain aspects of care, and measured actual contact time per patient category. The results showed a positive correlation with the dependency criteria. Using activity analyses, further studies were made of the activities of midwives, from which they were able to define more clearly the percentages of midwife time which were spent upon indirect care (27 per cent) and associated work (8.2 per cent) making direct care 64.8 per cent of total midwife time averaged out over all cases. This compares with Ball's assessment of 85 per cent for all direct and indirect care.

■ Other developments in measuring midwifery workload

☐ Using standard times for assessing midwifery workload

The preliminary findings of a standard time per activity method have been reported by Maclean and Bowden (1989). Nursing care plans were used to define patient needs, and locally produced quality of care standards provided specific criteria to describe different interventions needed by mothers and babies in postnatal wards. A very attractive and easy to complete score sheet was produced by which midwives could indicate the number and types of interventions required for each mother/baby dyad on each shift. Rather like the Grasp system (Meyer 1984), each intervention had a score which reflected the number of midwife care points needed. For example, changing a nappy was assessed as needing one midwife care point, but assisting a mother with breastfeeding needed 10 midwife care points. A working group of midwives, tutors and managers had estimated that one midwife care point required six minutes of midwife time to complete. On this basis therefore changing a nappy would require six minutes of midwife time on each occasion a nappy was changed, whereas each occasion of assisting breastfeeding would need 60 minutes per shift. The score sheet does not allow for more than one occurrence of each activity to be scored per shift, and one wonders whether this was found to be sufficient in use. The total midwife care points scored for each day per client forms the basis for assessing midwife time required. This neat, easy to use system was in its early stages at the time of publication.

☐ Using dependency based methods

Further work has been undertaken in Trent Region on developing dependency based workload measures for antenatal and postnatal care, both in hospital and the community (Trent Health 1991; Washbrook 1991).

■ Implications for clinical practice in the light of currently available evidence

The need to develop robust measures of workload is likely to increase as costing systems are developed for maternity care. These systems are also needed to provide information about the effectiveness and efficiency of the work of midwives. As has been discussed, these developments are in an early phase in midwifery practice, but the research already emerging is raising issues about care policies and practices in maternity care and helping midwives and obstetricians to make better decisions about the management of client care.

There is need however for much more research before the full picture of midwifery activity can be presented. Very little work has been done in community midwifery or in neonatal care. Designing workload measures and collecting and analysing data is time consuming and fraught with problems, some of which have been outlined in this chapter. The work already undertaken indicates that it is possible to measure midwifery workload in a valid way, and the development of quality assurance tools (All Wales Nurse Manpower Planning Committee 1985; Hughes & Goldstone 1990a, b, c) provides invaluable assistance in the research process.

Rhetoric is no longer sufficient. Midwives must back up their professional opinions of the needs of clients with sound information and discussion. The ability to debate and demonstrate the validity of one's decisions is a crucial component of good quality care management. The foundations have been laid and provide an excellent basis for further development.

■ Practice check

- How much does the workload fluctuate in your unit? Do you know what is the lowest and the highest number of births per day?

- Can you identify events or situations which create heavier than normal workload? If you can, would you consider that these are unavoidable, or could they be prevented with better planning?

- What are the criteria used to determine staff ratios in the place where you work? If these exist, do you consider that they are useful?

- How often do you feel that other demands prevent you from giving the kind of care you believe is needed by the client? Can you identify what these demands are? Could they be undertaken by clerical staff or by health care assistants?

- How would you measure the quality of the care you give? What criteria would you set? Discuss your answers with a colleague to see if you can reach a consensus together.

- What are the criteria used for setting staff rotas? Are the same number of staff deployed each day or shift? Are rotas set according to staff requests for time off? How much does the rota system assist or detract from continuity of care?

● Is flexitime used in your unit? If so, do you consider that this is good use of staff resources?

● How appropriate do you think it is for midwives to be attached to ward rotas? Could team work make it more possible to follow through the care of individual clients? Are there any difficulties in working within team midwifery?

■ References

All Wales Nurse Manpower Planning Committee (Midwifery Sub-group) 1985 Standards of care. HMSO, London

Audit Commission 1991 The virtue of patients: making the best use of ward nursing resources. HMSO, London

Auld M 1976 How many nurses? A method of estimating the requisite nursing establishment for a hospital. RCN, London

Ball J A, Goldstone L A, Collier M 1984 Criteria for care: the manual of the North West nurse staffing levels project. Newcastle Polytechnic Products Ltd, Newcastle upon Tyne

Ball J A, Oreschnik R 1986a Criteria for care. Senior Nurse 5 (4): 26–9

Ball J A, Oreschnik R 1986b Balanced formula. Senior Nurse 5 (5): 30–32

Ball J A 1987 A quality environment. Senior Nurse 5 (6): 23–4

Ball J A, Hurst K, Booth M, Franklin R 1989 But who will make the beds? Nuffield Institute and Mersey RHA, Leeds

Ball J A 1988 Dependency levels in the delivery suite. Proceedings of the Research and the Midwife Conference 1988

Ball J A 1989 Birth Rate: a method for outcome review and manpower planning for delivery suites. Nuffield Institute for Health Services Studies, Leeds

Ball J A 1992 Birth Rate using clinical indicators for assessing workload, staffing and care outcomes: an extended and revised edition of the original Birthrate manual. Nuffield Institute for Health Services Studies, Leeds

Barr A 1967 Measurement of nursing care. Oxford Regional Hospital Board, Oxford

Barr A, Moores B 1972 Nursing dependency as a basis for staff deployment. Oxford Regional Hospital Board, Oxford

Barr A, Moores B, Rhys Hearn C 1973 A review of the various methods of measuring the dependency of patients on nursing staff. International Journal of Nursing Studies 10: 195–208

Barr A 1984 Hospital nursing establishments and costs. Hospital and Health Service Review January: 31–7

Bell A, Storey C 1984 Assessing workload by a nursing study. Nursing Times 80 (34): 57–9

Boxall J, Garcia J 1983 Stress and the nurse in neonatal units. Midwives Chronicle 96 (1151): 409

British Paediatric Association and the Royal College of Obstetricians and Gynaecologists 1977 Recommendations for the improvement of infant care during the perinatal period in the UK: a discussion document. BPA/RCOG, London

British Paediatric Association and the Royal College of Obstetricians and Gynaecologists 1982 Midwife and nurse staffing and training for special care and the intensive care of the newborn: a consultative document. BPA/ RCOG, London

Brown C, Dawson J 1989 Calculating labour ward services: the art of the possible. Journal of Advanced Nursing 4: 559–68

Department of Health and Social Security 1980 The Second Report from the Social Services Committee on Perinatal and Neonatal Mortality. HMSO, London

Department of Health and Social Security 1983 Nurse Manpower Planning: Approaches and Techniques. HMSO, London

Gillett J, Flux R 1987 Acting on information. Nursing Times 83 (15):

Gillies D A 1982 Nursing management: a systems approach. W B Saunders, Philadelphia

Giovannetti P 1984 Staffing methods – implications for quality. In Willis L D, Linwood M E (eds) Measuring the quality of care. Churchill Livingstone, Edinburgh

Goddard H A 1963 Work measurement as a basis for calculating nursing establishments. Leeds Regional Hospital Board, Leeds

Goldstone L A, Ball J A, Collier M 1983 Monitor: an index of the quality of nursing care for acute medical and surgical wards. Newcastle Polytechnic Products Ltd, Newcastle upon Tyne

Grant N 1979 Time to care: a method of calculating nursing workload based on individualised patient care. RCN, London

Hilton I, Dawson J 1988 Monitor and Criteria for Care: the Portsmouth experience. Senior Nurse 8 (67): 26–8

Hughes D J F, Goldstone L A 1990 Midwifery Monitor I: pregnancy care. An audit of the quality of midwifery care in pregnancy Poly Enterprises Ltd, Leeds

Hughes D J F, Goldstone L A 1990 Midwifery Monitor II: labour care. An audit of the quality of midwifery care in labour. Poly Enterprises Ltd, Leeds

Hughes D J F, Goldstone L A 1990 Midwifery Monitor II: Care after the birth. An audit of the quality of postnatal midwifery care. Poly Enterprises Ltd, Leeds

Intensive Care Society 1985 Staffing for intensive care units. Intensive Care Society, London

Jelinek R C, Zinn T, Brya J 1973 Tell the computer how sick the patients are and it will tell you how many nurses they need. Modern Hospital 1973 (December): 81–5

Jelinek R C, Haussman R K D, Hegyvary S T, Newman J F 1974 A methodology for measuring quality of nursing. DHEW Publication No. (HRA) 76–25. USA Government Printing Office, Washington DC

Jelinek R C, Dennis L C 1976 A review and evaluation of nursing productivity. DHEW Publication No. (HRA) 77–70. USA Government Printing Office, Bethesda, Maryland

Jelinek R C, Haussman R K D, Hegyvary S T 1977 Monitoring quality of nursing care. Part 3: Professional review for nursing; an empirical investigation. DHEW Publication No. (HRA) 77–70. USA Government Printing Office, Washington DC

Knaus W A, Zimmerman J E, Wager D P, Draper E A, Lawrence D E 1982 APACHE – Acute Physiology and Chronic Health Evaluation: a physiologically based classification system. Critical Care Medicine 9: 591–7

Lelean S R 1976 Ready for report nurse? A study of nursing communication in hospital wards. RCN, London

Maclean G, Bowden H I 1989 Developing a midwifery workload management system: a preliminary report. Midwifery 5: 172–81

Maternity Services Advisory Committee 1985 Maternity Care in Action Part II. Care during childbirth (intrapartum care). HMSO, London

Meyer D 1984 Manpower planning: one American approach. Nursing Times 80 (34): 52–4

Morgan C J 1986 Severity scoring in intensive care. British Medical Journal 292: 1546

National Audit Office 1985 National Health Service: control of nursing manpower. Report of the comptroller and auditor general. HMSO, London

Pittman A 1991 Neonatal units: a review of the literature, with special emphasis on nursing and nurse staffing. Department of Nursing Studies, Queens Medical Centre, Nottingham

Reid N G, Melaugh M 1988 Nursing hours per patient: a method for allocation of staff in midwifery. International Journal of Nursing Studies 25 (1): 53–66

Royal College of Physicians 1988 Medical care of the newborn in England and Wales. RCP, London: 31

Rhys Hearn C 1974 Evaluation of patients' nursing needs: prediction of staffing. Occasional Papers 1, 2, 3 & 4. Nursing Times 70: 69–84

Scottish Home and Health Department 1969 Nursing workload as a basis for staffing: Report by Work Study Department of the North Eastern Regional Hospital Board. SSHD, Edinburgh

Senior O 1979 Dependency and establishments: A study of general hospital wards – the changeover from a non-teaching to a teaching hospital. RCN, London

Trent Health 1991 Report of the Trent Midwifery Manpower Planning Project. Trent RHA, Sheffield

Washbrook M 1991 Midwives and manpower – the means to examine our resources. MIDIRS Midwifery Digest 1991 (3): 259–61

■ Suggested further reading

Ball J A 1992 Birth Rate *** Using clinical indicators for assessing workload, staffing and care outcomes: an extended and revised edition of the original Birthrate manual. Available from Nuffield Institute for Health Services Studies, Leeds University, 71–75 Clarendon Road, Leeds LS2 9PL

Ball J A, Flint C, Garvey M, Jackson-Baker A, Page L 1992 Who's left holding the baby? An organisational framework for making the most of midwifery resources. Available from Nuffield Institute for Health Services Studies, Leeds University, 71–75 Clarendon Road, Leeds LS2 9PL

Maclean G, Bowden H I 1989 Developing a midwifery workload management system: a preliminary report. Midwifery 5: 172–81

Pittman A 1991 Neonatal units: a review of the literature with special emphasis on nursing and nurse staffing. Department of Nursing Studies, University of Nottingham

Washbrook M 1991 Midwives and manpower – the means to examine our resources. MIDIRS Midwifery Digest 1991 (3): 259–61

Chapter 10

Negligence litigation research and the practice of midwifery

Robert Dingwall

From a purely legal point of view, the delivery of babies is one of the most complicated areas of medical practice. Midwives and doctors share a monopoly over the right to attend a woman in childbirth. If anything goes wrong, however, they are uniquely vulnerable to being sued: childbirth is the only area of health care where most clinical actions simultaneously affect two potential plaintiffs! The risk of litigation has increased in recent years and some people think this has had an adverse effect on clinical practice. This trend has, in particular, been blamed for an increasing use of high technology interventions. These are said to be motivated by a desire to lay the basis of a legal defence for the birth attendant rather than by the wishes or interests of mothers and their babies. This is a questionable assertion but it has been important in the inter-professional politics of midwifery and obstetrics.

Unlike the other chapters in this book, no previous knowledge of the field is assumed. It begins by explaining the main ideas of negligence liability as a legal concept and then reviews recent research on its effects in the field of obstetric care. For reasons to be explained shortly, there is very little literature which deals specifically with the position of midwives in the United Kingdom, but the principles established from studies of obstetrics can be applied because, from a legal point of view, the context of practice is similar. Finally, the implications for policy and practice will be examined.

The discussion which follows is based on English law. At this level of generality, most of the points would apply to most Western legal systems but there are, of course, important differences in terminology and detail which would affect any particular example in any particular country.

■ What is 'negligence'?

Negligence actions against health care providers arise under the common law of tort. *Tort* is an old legal word which means a wrongdoing. There are several different kinds of tort, but we are concerned here with the tort of negligence. This rests on the assumption that members of a community have a duty to behave with reasonable care in the way they deal with each other. If I fail in this duty and my failure results in an injury to you, then you are entitled to seek compensation from me for any economic losses that you have incurred and for the general upset that you have experienced. The fact that I may have to compensate you for my neglect also creates an incentive for me to be careful in the way I deal with you. I must assess whether the possible benefits from taking a risk or cutting a corner are likely to be outweighed by the losses that I would suffer if my gamble did not succeed and I had to compensate for you some injury. In that situation, a court hearing and judgement might also send a signal to other people about the consequences of actions like mine and cause them to think more carefully before taking such risks themselves. The legal action may also have psychological benefits for you if you feel that I have been punished for my fault or, alternatively, that someone impartial has tested the facts and found that no wrong was committed. These four general objectives of tort litigation are often summarised as:

- Compensation;
- Deterrence;
- Inquiry;
- Retribution.

The person who brings a tort action for negligence, the plaintiff, has to prove two things against the defendant – *causation* and *fault*.

☐ Causation

This means that the defendant's actions have caused, or have made a material contribution to causing, the plaintiff's loss. Causation is often a difficult issue in medical cases. Medicine involves a complicated set of interactions between the physical condition of a patient, a therapeutic intervention and a complex social organisation of carers. Take vaccine damage as an example. There is a very small risk that pertussis vaccine can cause adverse reactions leading to irreversible brain damage. If this happens, how, in an individual case, do you decide whether a reaction following vaccination is causally related to the vaccination rather than just coincidental? Many children have fits because of illnesses, injuries or other random natural causes. Some of those fits lead to brain damage. In order to bring a successful lawsuit, the child or the adult bringing the action on their behalf, would have to prove that a particular fit could not have been a chance event that just happened to occur shortly after a vaccination. This is quite a stringent test and many medical claims fall at this first hurdle.

In some circumstances, a special rule of evidence called *res ipsa loquitur* (a Latin phrase meaning 'the thing speaks for itself') can weaken this requirement. Suppose that all the children vaccinated at a particular clinic on a particular day developed adverse reactions. The court can decide that this is so strongly suggestive of a defective batch of vaccine that the manufacturers should be liable, unless they can show that there was some other intervening cause. Perhaps the doctor was using a contaminated batch of needles to give the injections, in which the case the responsibility would lie with the suppliers or possibly with the staff responsible for infection control procedures in the clinic.

☐ **Fault**

Even if you can show a causal link between the intervention, or non-intervention, of a health care provider and an adverse outcome, this is not sufficient to prove that a wrong has been done. The tort of negligence deals in questions of fault. It is not intended as a general scheme for compensating victims of misfortune. So I am only liable to make some reparations to you if your injuries result from some failure on my part. In some areas, the law has established a principle of 'strict liability'. This means that my responsibility is so clear that there can be no way of escaping it. Suppose I buy and drink a bottle of milk contaminated with alkali and suffer chemical damage to my gastrointestinal tract. Even if it were not possible to show exactly how the contamination occurred, a court might decide that no dairy should organise its business in such a way that contamination of this kind could ever be possible. The dairy would be strictly liable for the purity of its milk.

The principle of strict liability is becoming more important because of directives from the European Community. Manufacturers are to be held liable for personal injuries arising from defects in their products that appear in the first 10 years after the product comes on the market. This principle could be quite important for pharmaceutical manufacturers, because it would mean that they would be clearly liable for any injuries caused by side effects of their products. However, in the United Kingdom, the principle has been weakened by the 'state of the art defence'. This means that a manufacturer's liability only extends to those risks that were foreseeable in the light of the scientific and technical knowledge at the time the product was developed. For example, this would not have helped the victims of the teratogenic effects of thalidomide, because the possibility of such deformities resulting from taking medication during pregnancy was not clearly recognised when the drug was being developed. There has been some discussion in the European Commission about extending strict liability to professional services but this has not yet been accepted.

Midwives also need to be aware of another version of strict liability, namely *breach of statutory duty*. If an Act of Parliament, or regulations made under an Act, says that I should act in a particular fashion and I fail to do so, then I may be found negligent just because I have failed to carry out my legal duty. If a midwife acts in a way that is contrary to the Midwives' Rules and injures a woman or her child, then she is likely to be found negligent, whatever her motives or reasons for breaking the rules. The breach alone is sufficient to create the tort.

At present, the liability of doctors is determined by what is usually called the *Bolam* principle after the 1957 case in which it was laid out. This sets a standard of care by reference to the 'practice accepted as proper by a responsible body of medical men skilled in that particular art'. This does not mean that a doctor has to do what every doctor would have done in a particular case, simply that there has to be a respectable body of opinion that his, or her, actions were reasonable in the circumstances. The qualification about skill is important. A doctor who takes on a case cannot excuse a lapse by claiming inexperience or inappropriate skills: if the doctor is presented with a problem requiring expertise, his or her work will be judged against the standard of those who have such knowledge and skill. There have been several cases where health authorities have been found negligent because of their failure to provide adequate senior cover to SHOs in areas like obstetrics. The junior doctors have taken on work beyond their level, often in emergencies, but this has been judged by the standard expected of the consultant or senior registrar who should have been available. This, of course, is an important pressure on employers to make sure that there is adquate staffing in acute areas of health care.

It is also important to note that the law recognises the concept of the non-negligent error. Because of the elements of judgement in medical practice, it is possible for clinicians to make reasonable decisions that turn out to be wrong and for which they should not be faulted. Without fault, there can be no negligence.

■ Alternatives to tort

Because tort litigation is based on the two tests of cause and fault, rather than on the needs of the injured person, it can produce many inequities. As a Royal College of Physicians Working Party noted, a child suffering brain damage because of obstetric mismanagement might collect £500 000–£750 000, a child suffering similar injury following vaccination may collect £20 000 under a statutory scheme and a child damaged by the complications of meningitis, correctly diagnosed and treated, may receive nothing (RCP 1990). All three children have the same needs for care but very different resources to meet them. For this reason, some countries have replaced the tort system by other means of compensating the victims of medical injuries. One set of schemes, in countries like Sweden, Finland and New Zealand, involve the creation of a special fund to pay compensation without the need to prove that someone was at fault. They are, consequently, known as *no-fault* systems. There is, however, still some inequity, in that they do not cover people who have similar conditions resulting from natural causes. This has led some people to argue instead for the general improvement of social security and welfare benefits and the provision of a *comprehensive disability income* (see, for example, Lamb and Percival 1992). Other theoretical solutions are reviewed by Ham *et al* (1988).

The Royal College of Physicians report lists several other weaknesses in the system. Of particular importance is its weakness as a means of exposing poor practice. In the nature of the system, clear cut cases are settled by negotiation with little publicity. The doctors who are exposed to public scrutiny are those who are operating in areas where there is a genuine difference of clinical opinion, where practice has evolved between the time of the incident and the time of the claim or where there is considerable uncertainty about the facts of the alleged behaviour. As a result, the professionals who do end up in court tend to be seen by their colleagues as unlucky rather than culpable. This severely dilutes both the deterrent and the standard setting aspects of the tort system. The report discusses the ways in which professional accountability might be improved alongside any possible reforms of patient compensation.

■ Midwives and negligence

There is very little modern case-law which deals specifically with negligent actions by midwives. This is because, since 1948, almost all practising midwives have been covered by the *vicarious liability* of their employer. This is a form of liability where an employer takes responsibility for the actions of employees within the scope of their employment. It is designed partly to ensure that victims of injury can recover compensation from someone who has a 'deeper pocket' and is better able to meet their claim and partly to discourage employers from putting their staff in positions where they must take risks or incur sanctions from managers or supervisors. Since then, any negligence by an NHS midwife has resulted in an action against her employing authority. The employer has a theoretical right to bring her into the case as an individual and to try to recover any payments from her. As far as I can establish, this right has never been exercised by the NHS. Although the right has passed to NHS Trusts, the Department of Health has also tried to discourage them from making use of it (Personal communication, but see, DoH 1989 and NHS Management Executive 1990).

Within the NHS, however, the doctors thought that it was important that they should continue to influence the way litigation was handled. They feared that NHS authorities might deal with cases on a simple economic basis so that some claims could be settled purely because it was cheaper to pay than to fight. Where a doctor's professional reputation was at stake, such a policy could have considerable personal costs, in that a settlement, even without an admission of liability, was likely to damage his or her standing with patients or peers. At a rather later point, the fear was also expressed that health authorities might be less willing to pursue what were essentially test cases for a new technique or mode of practice where the costs of the individual action might be quite disproportionate to the losses alleged, encouraging settlement, but where the implications for the profession as a whole might be considerable. From 1954 until 1990, then, liability was shared between health authorities and employed doctors. The authorities and the medical defence organisations, who insured the doctors, would agree between themselves how the costs of defending or settling a case should be divided, according to their estimate of how far the alleged harm was caused by the doctors involved and how far it resulted from the actions of other NHS staff. A birth injury caused by improper use of forceps would result in all the costs falling on the defence organisation, while an injury resulting from a midwife failing to notice that a monitor was faulty would be a cost to the health authority.

This system broke down under the pressures from the rising costs and numbers of negligence actions in the 1980s and was replaced by a form of employers' liability for the actions of doctors. Although there are some technical differences, all NHS employees are now covered by essentially the same legal arrangements, with the main costs falling on their employers, currently provider units and NHS Trusts. (GPs, as independent contractors, have always been and remain individually liable.)

This has been quite important in terms of inter-professional relations, because obstetricians used to be individually liable for the outcome of their care of a patient in a way midwives in NHS practice were not. Many obstetricians thought that this should give them a special voice in the determination of unit policies. While this argument is now less valid, there are still significant differences in the midwives' position. The most important of these comes from the *Bolam* standard of care. Where the work of midwives and obstetricians overlaps, it seems likely that the standard will still be set by reference to that endorsed by doctors rather than by midwives so as to discourage employers from indiscriminate substitution of midwives for doctors. There will, for example, be only one standard set for the decision to perform an episiotomy and one quality of repair, whoever carries it out. A midwife performing this task must do so to the standard of an averagely skilful obstetrician rather than to some other standard set in relation to the skills, experience and training of midwives. This would be equally true for a midwife in independent practice.

■ Obstetric litigation in the United Kingdom

The general increase in litigation about medical negligence in the United Kingdom since the early 1980s is widely thought to have had a particularly damaging effect on the practice of obstetrics. In reality, the picture is a good deal more complicated than the bare statistics might suggest and the evidence of harm is more ambiguous than some commentaries on this trend might lead us to think.

Obstetrics and gynaecology cases certainly contribute a significant proportion of the negligence claims brought against the NHS. In a study of the 470 traceable closed claims against District Health Authorities in the Oxford Region between 1974 and 1988, it was found that 22 per cent of the claims originated from this specialty (Dingwall & Fenn 1991). However, they represented only 16.7 per cent of the successful claims and 8.8 per cent of the total loss, the aggregate of costs and damages paid out by the authorities. For this Region in this period, obstetric and gynaecological claims had a lower than average success rate and where payments were made, they were relatively small. The series chanced not to include any major cases based on allegations of serious 'brain damage' and was, in fact, dominated by relatively low value gynaecological cases. This finding, though, is consistent with the indications that major obstetric claims were only being opened at a rate of 50–100 per year in the United Kingdom throughout this period (Capstick & Edwards 1990; Acheson 1991). Even if recent changes in the legal aid rules, making it easier for children to sue, lead to an increase in the base rate to 200 opened claims per year, this would still only be one per district per year. Since the success rate seems to be around 25–30 per cent (Hawkins and Patterson 1987; Capstick & Edwards 1990; Dingwall & Fenn 1991) this suggests that the typical district will be hit with a big pay out just once every four years on average. Nationally, of course, the costs may be significant: the Medical Protection Society estimated that obstetric claims were accounting for 30 per cent of the total losses of the defence organisations at the point when liability was taken over by the NHS (Acheson 1991). A sense of perspective is important though: big obstetric cases are not an everyday phenomenon, although they can have major implications for defendants when they do occur.

How can this be reconciled with the gloom expressed by many obstetricians? Is litigation really having a big effect on the practice of obstetrics and the recruitment to the specialty? Three points seem important here.

First, there is no evidence that obstetrics has had a significantly different experience from the rest of the medical profession. There has been a temporary blip resulting from the changes in legal aid rules, which seem to have brought forward cases that would otherwise have had to wait until the child reached the age of 16 and was assessed on his or her own income and assets. This appears to have produced a bunching of claims – the Spastics Society (Lamb & Percival 1992) suggest that 600 were opened in 1991 – and we should expect the rate to stabilise as this effect works through. There might be a slight increase eventually, since some children will now file claims who might otherwise have died before they became eligible for legal aid, but this seems likely to be a small number. Overall, if anything, obstetrics' share of the total volume of negligence litigation may have declined slightly in the 1980s (Capstick & Edwards 1990). It is worth remembering, too, that most UK professions experienced an upsurge in negligence litigation in that decade (Ham *et al* 1988). Given this, it seems likely the explanation of the upward trend in litigation will involve factors that are not exclusive to the provision of health care. Similar conclusions have been reached from a recent study of Canadian experience (Dewees *et al* 1991). These might include some general decline in deference to professional authority, rising expectations of professional services, the fragility of the economy leaving disappointed clients less able to absorb losses and more vigorous marketing of legal services. There is, however, no conclusive evidence for the specific contribution of any of these to rising litigation rates.

Second, there is no convicing evidence that litigation has played more than a minor role in changing clinical practice. Caesarean section rates have increased world wide, both in 'high' litigation countries like the USA and England and 'low' litigation countries like Norway and The Netherlands (see Fig. 10.1).

More recent unpublished data from the Organisation for Economic Co-operation and Development for years around 1986 cited by Renwick (1991) show no association between litigation experience and rank order in an

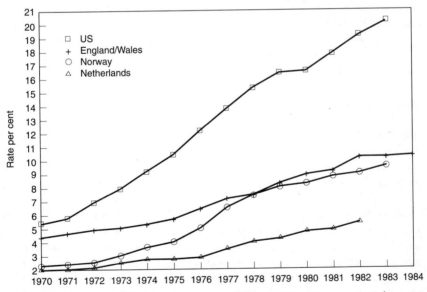

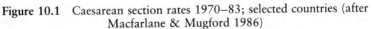

Figure 10.1 Caesarean section rates 1970–83; selected countries (after Macfarlane & Mugford 1986)

international league table of caesarean rates. The United Kingdom, for example, has a similar caesarean rate to New Zealand, which has effectively abolished tort litigation in favour of a mixture of no-fault and social security provision. The highest rates in Europe are found in Portugal, which is not known to have any significant amount of medical litigation. From an extensive review of international literature up to the late 1980s, Dingwall *et al* (1991) concluded that changes in caesarean section rates could be better explained by changing clinical indications, policies on repeat caesareans, time management advantages for both women and obstetricians and systems of reimbursement that made caesarean sections more profitable than vaginal deliveries. Further support for this analysis has come from a recent study of variations in caesarean rates within Australia by Renwick (1991) which finds a greater incidence among insured women living in State capitals and argues that this is related to the readier availability of obstetricians and the resources available to the women.

The claim that litigation has resulted in changes in practice rests mainly on anecdotal evidence, although there have been a few surveys conducted among obstetricians. The Maternity Alliance (1986) surveys in Britain are often held up as showing the association between litigation and caesarean section rates, while two surveys of members by the American College of Obstetricians and Gynecologists (ACOG 1983; 1985) are widely cited as evidence of more general changes in clinical practice. Such self-report studies on the effects of a single motivation should, however, be treated with great caution. They almost invariably lead to an overstatement of the impact of that motive relative to other possibilities (Danzon 1985). Most of the American findings, for example, can be as well explained by the changing economic context of practice (Dingwall *et al* 1991). Some reported changes might actually be thought to benefit women and children such as the closer observation, improved record keeping and greater use of second opinion reported in the ACOG surveys. An advocate for the tort system might say that this showed it working properly in inducing doctors to take greater care.

The same argument might be used about the reported abandonment of practice by obstetricians. In the North American context, for which more evidence is available, the pattern seems more easily explained by the marginal economic viability of medical care in poor and sparsely populated rural areas with ageing populations. The doctors who are giving up seem to be people with low volumes of practice and a lack of confidence in the currency of their skills (Dingwall *et al* 1991). Just as in the United Kingdom, the United States has long had a policy of trying to move obstetric care from small local units to regional centres (Hein 1986). The tort system is merely adding another pressure in favour of this policy by raising insurance rates to the point where marginal providers find it uneconomic to continue. The same pressure would apply to hospitals, if their insurance costs were as closely related to the risk of a claim (Luft *et al* 1991). There is an obvious policy dilemma here in the balance between the concentration of deliveries in centres where skills can be honed and kept sharp and specialised resources most economically provided, and the promotion of an accessible community service close to the homes of women and their families. Litigation, however, is a subsidiary factor in this debate, not its motor.

Finally, the argument that litigation is having a deterrent effect on recruitment seems inconsistent with what is known about the process of career choice and the variety of influences that determine the pursuit of one track rather than another (Johnson 1983). Again, the best evidence is American, but the annual surveys of specialty choices among graduating medical students have shown no evidence of any changes in the relative attractiveness of different specialties that could be associated with litigation rates (Institute of Medicine 1989). To the extent that there are problems in recruitment to obstetrics in the UK, they may have more to do with the gloomy comments of senior figures than the experience of the specialty.

■ Recommendations for clinical practice in the light of currently available information

The most important recommendation is not to panic. If your practice is based on sound research or clinical experience, is carefully documented and in accord with policies shared by the whole obstetric team, you have nothing to fear from negligence litigation. The most important reasons why health authorities have to pay out large sums for cases where the scientific evidence for a causal relationship between maternity care and adverse outcomes is weak, as in cerebral palsy, are that some aspect of the original practice is found to be indefensible or some key data are missing. The loss of a monitoring trace can cost £750 000 because it becomes impossible to prove that vital signs remained regular throughout delivery and to argue that a case of cerebral palsy should be considered as one of the 80–90 per cent that are now thought not to be associated with birth trauma (Lamb & Lang 1992). The legal process can also be a cruel exposure of failures in team work. If one professional group has adopted policies and practices at odds with those of the others, a plaintiff's lawyer will have a field day with the discrepancies. In effect, though, the objective of the tort system is to encourage good practice, so that, if your practice is soundly based, the result should not be a penalty for your employer.

Midwives in independent practice need to be particularly cautious. It is sometimes thought that they are less likely to be sued because they have a better relationship with their clients. This, however, is rather disingenuous. It seems more likely that they deal with a lower risk population. Anyhow, surely some questions should be asked about the morality of discouraging an injured patient from obtaining compensation to which she is entitled just because of a personal loyalty to her birth attendant. A child suffering some form of delivery trauma because of negligence has the same needs, whether delivered by a ham-fisted obstetrician or an over zealous natural midwife. At the least, there would seem to be a professional responsibility to carry an adequate level of insurance, not for the protection of the midwife but to ensure that injured clients can actually receive compensation that may be well in excess of her personal wealth.

There are, clearly, still important limitations on knowledge relating to the United Kingdom, especially in the context of midwifery, where the traditional division of labour in maternity care and the allocation of costs between the NHS and MDOs did not encourage service providers to treat research as a priority. The introduction of risk management philosophies to NHS services presents major challenges in its attempt to identify individual and organisational factors that are likely to achieve safe outcomes for both professionals and their clients (Vincent *et al* in press). There is also likely to be a continuing debate over the best way to compensate people who are injured by the negligent acts of health care professionals.

■ Discussion points

1. Would either no-fault or disability income support schemes be preferable to the tort system?

2. How would standards of care be affected if the punitive effects of tort were removed?

3. How could professional accountability be strengthened?

4. What are the best ways of explaining to 'patients' what has gone wrong?

5. How can professional and organisational learning from failures of care be promoted?

■ Practice check

• How good are your records from a legal point of view? Are they clearly written? Were they made at the time or as soon as reasonably practicable afterwards? Are there readings missing? Are entries by different people identified by name?

• Take some records made on your unit three or four years ago. How helpful are they? Can you tell who wrote what when? Are all the monitoring data and test results still there? Do you know where to find staff or students who have moved on since?

- Does your unit have a hotline for reporting adverse events so that all the evidence can be made secure and statements taken while everyone's memory is fresh? Can anyone use this? If you are in independent practice, does your insurer offer a similar service? Should you have your own legal consultant to provide this service?

- Is practice in your unit based on clearly stated policies and procedures? Who contributes to these? Are they based on well founded and up to date research evidence? How are these policies monitored and enforced? If you are in independent practice, how could you show that your knowledge was current and valid?

- Do you regularly attend or get feedback from local perinatal mortality and morbidity meetings? Are adverse events carefully reviewed by a multidisciplinary group and the results fed back to all the groups involved? If you are in independent practice, how could you show that your problems and difficulties had been reviewed by someone else and that you had learned from them?

■ References

Acheson D 1991 Law suit crisis poses threat to obstetric care. Hospital Doctor   C11: 12

American College of Obstetricians and Gynecologists 1983 Professional liability insurance and its effects: report of a survey of American College of Obstetricians and Gynecologists' membership. ACOG, Washington DC

American College of Obstetricians and Gynecologists 1985 Professional liability and its effect: report of a survey of American College of Obstetricians and Gynecologists' membership. ACOG, Washington DC

Capstick J B, Edwards P J 1990 Medicine and the law: trends in obstetric malpractice claims. Lancet   336: 931–2

Danzon P 1985 Medical malpractice. Harvard University Press, Cambridge, Mass

Department of Health 1989 Health Circular HC (89) 34. Claims of medical negligence against NHS hospital and community doctors and dentists. DoH, London

Dewees D N, Trebilcock M J, Coyle P C 1991 The medical malpractice crisis: a comparative empirical perspective. Law and Contemporary Problems   54 (1): 217–51

Dingwall R, Fenn P 1991 Is risk management necessary? International Journal of Risk and Safety in Medicine   2: 91–106

Dingwall R, Fenn P, Quam L 1991 Medical negligence: a review and bibliography. Centre for Socio-Legal Studies, Oxford

Ham C, Dingwall R, Fenn P, Harris D R 1988 Medical negligence: compensation and accountability. Kings Fund Institute/Centre for Socio-Legal Studies, London/Oxford

184 · *Midwifery Practice 4*

Hawkins C, Patterson I 1987 Medicolegal audit in the West Midlands region: analysis of 100 cases. British Medical Journal 295: 1533–6

Hein H N 1986 The status and future of small maternity services in Iowa. Journal of the American Medical Association 255: 1899–903

Institute of Medicine 1989 Medical professional liability and the delivery of obstetric care. National Academy of Sciences, Washington, DC

Johnson M 1983 Professional careers and biographies. In Dingwall R, Lewis P (eds) The sociology of the professions: lawyers, doctors and others. Macmillan, London

Lamb B, Percival R 1992 Paying for disability – no fault compensation: panacea or Pandora's Box? Spastics Society, London

Lamb B, Lang R 1992 Aetiology of cerebral palsy. British Journal of Obstetrics and Gynaecology 99: 176–8

Lutf H S, Katz P P, Pinney D G 1991 Risk factors for hospital malpractice exposure: implications for managers and insurers. Law and Contemporary Problems 54 (2): 43–64

Macfarlane A, Mugford M 1986 An epidemic of caesareans. Journal of Maternal and Child Health 11: 38–42

Maternity Alliance 1986 One birth in nine. Maternity Alliance, London

NHS Management Executive 1990 Executive letter EL(90) 191: Handling Claims of medical negligence

Renwick M Y 1991 Caesarean section rates, Australia 1986: variations at state and small area level. Australia and New Zealand Journal of Obstetrics and Gynaecology 31 (4): 299–304

Royal College of Physicians 1990 Compensation for adverse consequences of medical intervention. RCP, London

Vincent C, Ennis M, Audley R in press. Medical accidents. Oxford University Press, Oxford

■ Suggested further reading

Harlow C 1987 Understanding tort law. Fontana, London

Dingwall R, Fenn P (eds) 1992 Quality and regulation in health care. Routledge, London

Harvard Medical Practice Study 1990 Patients, doctors and lawyers: medical injury, malpractice litigation and patient compensation in New York. Harvard Medical Practice Study, New York

Index